MORTAL KARATE

No more competition

Self defense for the whole family
By Master Leonardo Gudiño

攻心為上　攻城為次　攻人為下

Authentic Military Karate
AND
Self defense

Illustrations: Shifu Leonardo Gudiño (TobiSpartan)

Rights Reserved according to the law.

Origin Mexico.

Quántóu Yata no Karasu
(Translated as Fist of the Eight-feathered Raven)

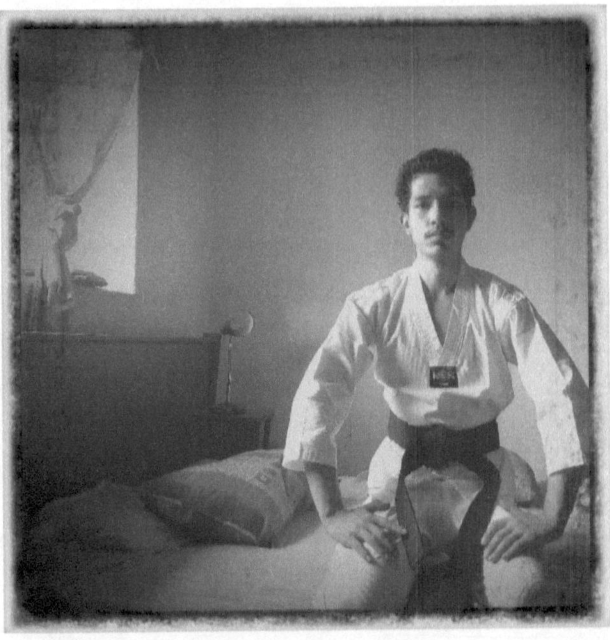

Shifu Leonardo Gudiño is a martial artist, philosopher, and draftsman; practitioner of the Wing Chun style, and the founder of his style of Huáng Lóng Kung Fu which contains three main styles the Raven style of "MORTAL KARATE" the Tiger style of "TIGER BOXING" and the Dragon style in "EL DRAGON HUANGLONG KUNG FU "which seeks to show real rapid defense techniques, along with a philosophy, ideology and approach, as well as giving the warrior freedom to continue adding skills or techniques to his repertoire.

Foreword:

Where exactly Karate was born and who invented it are data that are lost in the mists of time; it is only known with precision that it is a martial art, born of the need to defend oneself, using as the only weapons, the natural ones with which we have been endowed by mother nature; arms and legs, which, through special forms of training, become unique combat elements, to attack vulnerable points of the human being.

Karate means in its literal translation, "empty hand"; had its cradle in Asia, where the traditional patience and observation technique, made of something non-existent a true science of the art of self defense; Such science was the secret heritage of family clans that jealously passed on from generation to generation, their extraordinary knowledge. Hence, Karate, although the same deep down, has different projections depending on where it is learned.

To present it to my readers, in this modest treatise, I have compiled the most assimilable phases of this sport, in which sagacity, intelligence and cunning, rather than brute force, are determining factors. I consider and recommend Karate as the ideal sport for today's youth, since one of its healthy sporting performances is to provide its practitioners with a strong, agile body, resistant to all kinds of fatigue and efforts, creating a healthy and tenacious mind. , in addition to a vigorous spirit of improvement.

The companionship and courage. It stimulates chivalry, allowing a healthy vent to the innate warlike inclinations of the young; Only the astonishing diligence, energy, perseverance and intelligence of the Orientals could unite to offer the world the fruits of this wonderful sport and exceptional system of personal defense.

In this treatise I present a type of Karate, functional, since it eliminates those difficult to assimilate or dangerous sets, adapting them to modern training means, which deviate somewhat from the canons of pure classism, but which in their final results facilitate their teaching and training.

I wish and I hope that this treatise will be useful to my readers and that they will grasp the beautiful message of effort, discipline, improvement and chivalry, which is implicit in learning this beautiful sport.

Master Leonardo Gudiño

A healthy mind in a healthy body

Flower of Youth; Physical training.

Before learning to read and write, it is necessary to spell, know the alphabet, starting with the letter A and so on until you can read. This is precisely what we will do with the reader: We will take him by the hand, teaching him little by little, step by step, but without pause, in order to make him an expert karate and self-defense performer. We will start by preparing it physically.

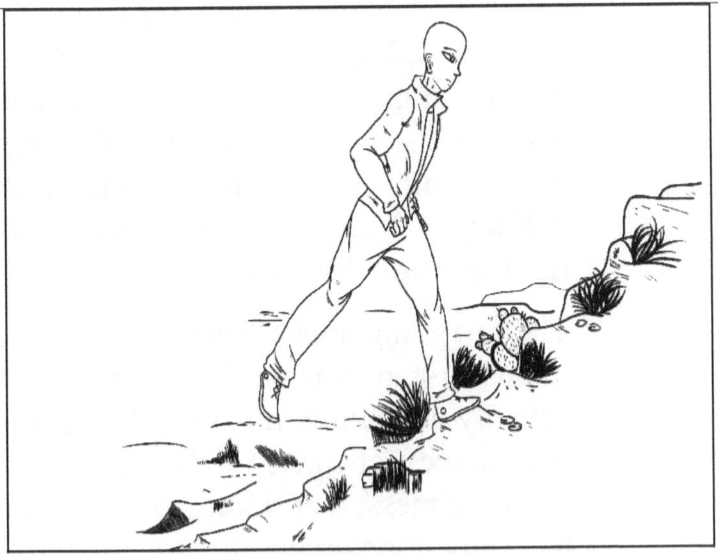

To do this, the applicant must request the approval of a doctor, through a thorough examination; Once this essential requirement is covered, we will enter into the matter.

The above with the sole purpose of letting the practitioner know about their body and if it has any genetic or functional limitations.

After getting to know your body physically, you need to adapt the exercises within your range, for example, if you cannot jump, do cardio, etc.

In some cases such as asthma, or injuries it is recommended to read "La Salud del Dragon" by the same author.

The sport that we are now trying to get to know, one hundred percent manly, requires, apart from maximum muscular performance, a solid resistance to the considerable effort required by the training necessary for learning; therefore, we will begin to toughen it up by subjecting it to a rigid sporting discipline.

The foregoing about "manly" is to indicate that in this case, as it is not for sporting purposes but actually defending, it is intended to have in preference a character and desire to gain strength and toughness, therefore, women should not have any impediment for reasons aesthetic, weight, taste, or emotional.

Anyone who wants strength will find the exercises practical and correct for a body of iron; regardless of gender, age, or physical condition (the latter knowing how to match you).

As the first part of this training, there is cross country running, preferably in a place full of trees; This practice should be done every day, trying to cover a minimum of two kilometers, increasing the distance as your body effortlessly supports the route. The way indicated for running, should be slow and steady at first, without precipitation, breathing widely through the nose, naturally, with the mouth closed, without forcing; After the first five hundred meters of light jogging, do a fast route, of a hundred meters more or less, and then fall back into the slow and rhythmic run, in order to normalize the breathing; when it has recovered and after running another five hundred meters, it will rehearse a new "sprint" (short and fast race) of another hundred meters, to again fall into a light trot and so on until completing the quota of more or less two kilometers. When doing this practice, especially the first few days, you should not exert yourself, as the result can be counterproductive; try to find the ideal one without unnecessary forcing, thus preparing the lungs for subsequent workouts; During the run, carefully monitor your breathing, keep warm in a thick, closed sweatshirt.

After the previous race, we will move on to performing a series of calisthenic exercises that are illustrated on the following pages.

Each of these exercises should be done an average of fifteen to twenty times per session. My recommendation is to do the number of exercises that each reader feels good, according to their muscular conformation, since too many exercises, instead of beneficial, are detrimental, since they tighten the muscles too much, a negative thing in any sport, because A man with strong muscles is slow to move, which is not an advantageous situation, since what we need is speed and agility if we want to stand out as Katatists.

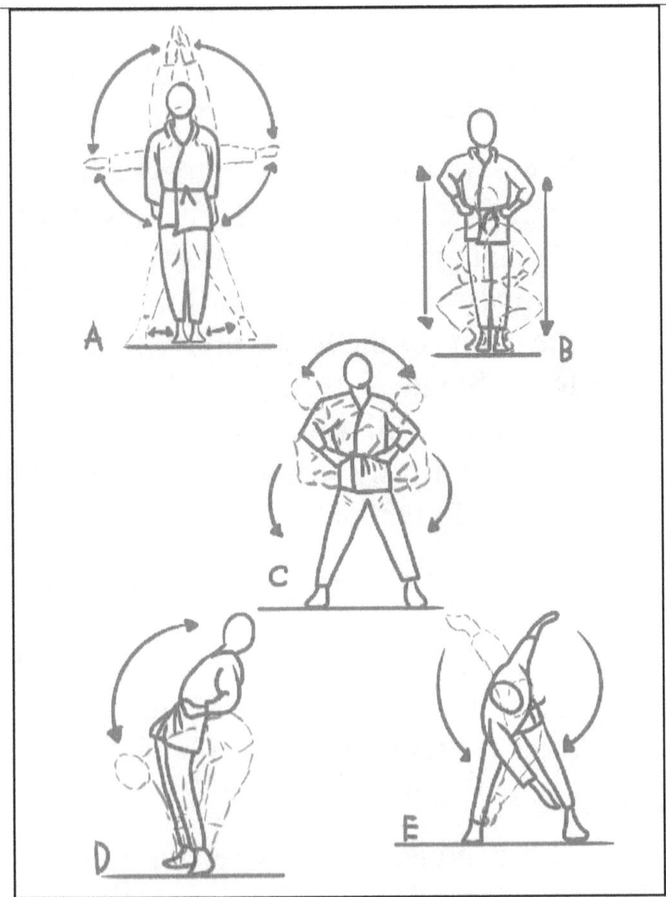

At this point, with the formal sports training, the reader will notice that his appetite improves significantly, having to take care of his diet based on abundant vegetables, eggs, meat and fish, avoiding as much as possible the ingestion of acid fats, flours, and in general , foods strong in acids, and calories; the sleep will be heavier and more restful, therefore try to sleep more; an average of 8 to 9 hours is advisable, or naps of 6 hours in the afternoon and night, to replace the wear and tear caused by training.

About more correct feeding information; the book "The health of the Dragon" is recommended.

Now, we will begin with the warm-up exercise marked with the letter A. It consists of: from standing to attention, jumping by opening the compass and at the same time giving a clap with the palms of the hands above the head, returning to the Stand at attention with another leap, then your arms will lower forcefully to their natural position, firmly striking your thighs with the palms of your hands.

The exercise marked with the letter B, is known to all as "squats"; We will do these by jumping to our feet, later standing on the tips of the feet, springing in order to stiffen the calves; from there we will go down with a lot of fiber and again we join with a jump.

This exercise is highly recommended to spring your legs. Run it about twenty times per session minimum.

Exercise C deals with rotating movements of the waist.

Apart from being a great method of avoiding the so-called "tires", it gives great elasticity and spring to the waist; you have to do twenty movements per side.

The one marked with the letter D, refers to exercises of bending the waist, it is very good to obtain spring: throw your body back, forcing the head as much as possible and from there touch the floor with the palms of the hands, keeping stiff legs; watch the drawing of the spring with the movements. Also run it twenty times per session.

Now we will go on to treat the exercise of the letter E, explained in the graph quite clearly. It is another exercise to give ease to the aspirant, to have spring. Force back the hand that is above, so that when you lower it you can do it easily; this exercise is highly recommended to reduce waistline. Like the previous ones, do it twenty times per session.

The exercise marked with the letter F on the page is a bit difficult for beginners, although of great value, as it provides extraordinary elasticity. Do this movement only ten times, practicing very carefully during the first few sessions. Don't overdo the note, seek help the first few times you practice it.

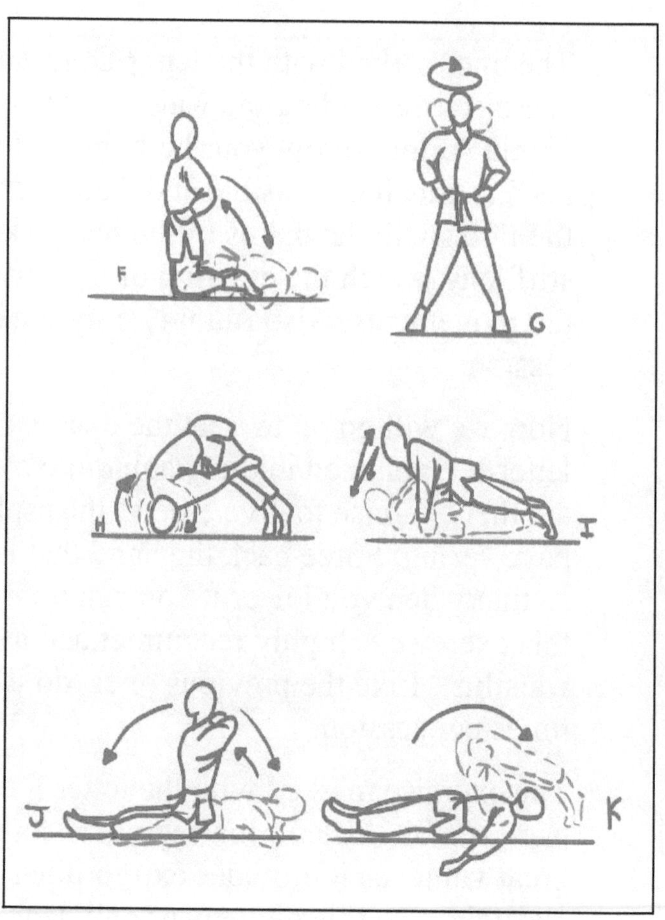

The marking with the letter G is self-explanatory. It is an exercise that tends to give lightness, ease and speed to the neck: make twenty turns to the right, and to get rid of the dizziness, do as many to the left, then back to front, sticking the beard on the chest. At the end of the series, loosen the neck with light movements for both sides.

The exercise indicated by the letter H is a bit rough, so it will not be practiced more than ten times.

It is the one indicated to harden the neck, and turn it, by strength, equal to that of a bull. The graph clearly indicates the exact pattern to follow.

The exercise of the letter I, is commonly known as "Push-ups", must be done twenty times; The first days we will do ten, but after the first week of work, we will increase the amount until we reach the indicated quota.

Try to do this exercise leaning on the tips of the fingers of the hands, in order to harden them; throw your head as far back as you can, trying to touch the ground with the tip of your beard; This is a fabulous exercise that for no reason should we stop practicing on a daily basis, as it is key to turning a man from a weakling.

Now we will go on to a very strong exercise, essential to harden one of the soft parts of the body, that is, the stomach; It is necessary to practice it a minimum of twenty times daily, doing it with great enthusiasm and fiber, touching the legs with the forehead, so that they are firmly seated on the floor, without bending the knee one millimeter.

To finish this series of exercises, we will do twenty movements equal to the one marked with the letter K, which serves as a rest to the previous one and complements it; gives a lot of strength to the soft parts, also providing athletic form to the aspirant, being also highly recommended to achieve spring. (I explain this in detail in the respective chapter.) I recommend that my readers write down their measurements in advance, taking a photograph of their body before starting this course, in order to compare the two three months later.

You will notice immediately that your body tends to become that of a perfect athlete, that your muscles have increased in toughness and strength, so that the aspirant will be ready to enter the rough training of sport, without fear of hurting himself, Well, in its current condition, it will withstand perfectly, without any hassle, Karate skirmishes, no matter how rough they are.

With all intention I left for the last a very simple practice, but of great value, which seems illustrated in the previous graph. As can be seen, it consists of walking quickly on a wooden crossbar placed at a certain height, doing it from front to back and vice versa, very quickly, standing on one foot and with the other executing imaginary kicks to the front, to the sides and back. . This exercise gives a lot of agility, balance, strength and security to the legs, it is the most recommended exercise that can exist for a good physical preparation.

The crossbar will be approximately four meters long, in case it cannot be achieved, intelligently replace it with a fence or something similar, which will allow you to achieve the wonderful performances derived from your training with your practice.

To finish your gym session, go around the room where you do your workouts, jumping with one leg, the other will carry up, alternate the leg when tired.

With the above, we will conclude this chapter, which is the most important of all, since, without its proper assimilation, it is not advisable to move on. The previous physical preparation must be very intense the first two or three months, then it will last the applicant's entire life, adapted to the exact type of sports routine that he wishes to carry out, but I insist, it should never be abandoned.

Well, taking for granted that the applicant has already worked three months on his physical preparation, we can enter into the matter.

I present to my readers this modern treatise on Karate and Self-defense, in which I have compiled all those sets, tricks and blows, which in my opinion are more assimilable for the Latin idiosyncrasy and temperament. The forms of training that I advise depart from the traditional oriental mysticism, but they redound to the benefit of the aspirant, who, with the theory in this book, receives extraordinary knowledge of Personal Defense. These are wonderful, practically unknown blows, in which, as the only weapons, parts of the body are used.

The most important thing is that insensibly they will become a magnificent sport, which will provide them, apart from a strong body and resistant muscles, great confidence in themselves; But I must remind my kind readers that in sports you only get success if you practice tirelessly, always correcting yourself, looking for better techniques, debugging mistakes and aiming at physical and mental improvement.

Our sport, although it is true that it gives us a great advantage over the profane in this knowledge, we must also recognize that it does not give us a clear letter of invulnerability, since there are people with whom we can stumble, who, without any sports education, They are capable of defeating anyone, be it because of their innate strength or their fighting spirit. Hence, because of the fact of reading or practicing well or badly what is written in these pages, they do not believe that they are invincible, on the contrary, we must never underestimate the contrary before knowing it, much less if we have perfectly well assimilated everything here tried, in addition to having many years of advantage shedding copious sweat in training.

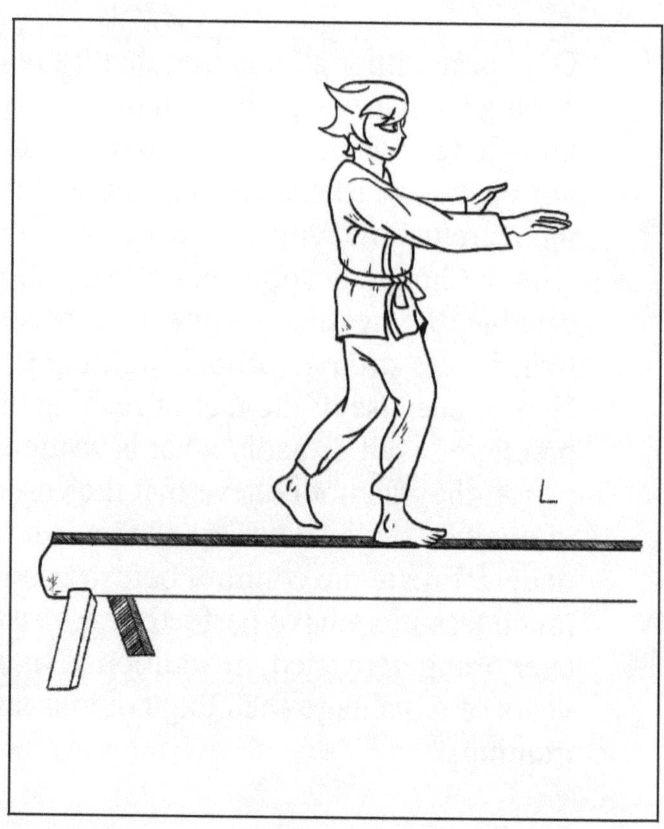

Our sport is a sport of long-term patient discipline; If we start today, let us bear in mind that in order to affirm that we half know it, it will be necessary to have practiced it tirelessly for many years, so that the reader thinks that, by acquiring this book, he is buying a life sentence of healthy recreation and sports improvement.

Mental Preparation

This treatise contains extremely crude hauls, the results of which can be disastrous, therefore, before entering fully into its learning, I beg my readers to reflect as necessary, mentally preparing themselves to receive extraordinary knowledge in their sporting performances, which will serve as a weapon for personal defense, but that by its own rudeness, is equivalent to bringing something more powerful than a firearm with a cut cartridge, recommending that irresponsibility, nervousness or lack of moral quality turn a beautiful sport into a danger to themselves or for their peers.

The knowledge of Karate and Self Defense that you will find here, should be considered as a healthy sport, of course for strong people, since it contains the equivalences of Boxing and Jiujitzu, sports that allow a decent outlet of the natural bellicose inclinations of young people and that at the same time they harden their muscles, preparing them properly to emerge gracefully from any contingency where it is essential to defend themselves.

Therefore, my readers must imbue their spirit and mind with nobility, decency and chivalry, to make this sport a means of physical improvement and moral toughness.

In practice and during the necessary skirmishes aimed at delving into the secrets of this treaty, a partner is needed, since otherwise it is not 100% practicable; It is in this case that we must most immerse ourselves in chivalry and sports self-denial, seeking healthy practices without hurting the partner, remembering the Olympic blazon that in sport, the main thing is not to win, but to compete and, in our case, to learn in every practice, both our victories and our defeats.

The second aspect to take care of, of capital importance, is serenity, since a karate performer must be a serene, calm man who does not let any emotion show on his face; his emotional control must be absolute during the development of the skirmishes, his face will be as cold and impenetrable as that of a statue, and he must not have nerves; This vital aspect is only acquired with constant practice and a rigid personal physical control of pain and emotions.

The third indispensable aspect to take care of, is to lose the fear of the blow; Well, although it is true that we learn how to cushion blows, it is also true that they hurt and much more in the early stages. This can lead to the applicant losing confidence and becoming afraid; Therefore, it is necessary that before having the first formal skirmish, he blanks himself with many days of intense physical preparation practice, with which, by increasing the strength of his muscles, he will also increase his confidence and serenity in the same way; confidence that will gradually increase as you gradually absorb the routine knowledge of formal sets, carefully put into practice.

Finally, I will deal with two aspects that are the key to success: Tenacity in your sports preparation and enthusiastic aggressiveness in casting.

The first is acquired with a constant and relentless discipline of daily training.

The second is natural in some people, but susceptible to develop in those who do not have it; This must be part of our training and mental preparation, a logical consequence of the confidence that is acquired with the constant skirmishes.

Therefore, I insist once again that it is necessary to take the physical and mental aspects of the aspirant by the hand in the practices, so that both, in their exact conjunction, lead him to success, a success that is not only observed in sport , but will happily transcend in all aspects of his life, in the life of an athlete who is healthy in body and mind, who will wear the following wise words as his coat of arms:

1. **TENACITY FOR LEARNING AND ITS PRACTICE**
2. **SUBLIMIZATION OF DETAIL AND CLASSICISM**
3. **SERENE AND CALCULATED AGGRESSIVENESS**
4. **SPORTS KNIGHT**

With the above elements and thirty minutes a day of training, all my readers will become, after a few years, extraordinary performers of this beautiful sport.

Special Recommendations

I recommend that my readers take due note of the following recommendations:

A. If the applicant does not feel in perfect physical condition, he should not accept for any reason to participate in any skirmish.

B. If during a practice it is necessary to stop it, in order to suit any of the contestants, an agreed signal will suffice for the practice to stop immediately. The signal can be oral or give three blows on the opponent's body; This is a pact between gentlemen and athletes, which must be respected to the letter.

C. In the event that a KO is raised during any training session, the applicant must take a week off before accepting a new skirmish; it is certainly advisable to visit a doctor asking for his opinion about the accident.

D. Do not skirmish after eating or during the digestion process.

E. It is not convenient to practice with novices who do not yet know the principles of defense; Train with experts to guide, protect, and teach you.

F. Do not confuse machismo with what prudence advises.

G. Make sport as broad a cult as a religion. Remember that the knowledge in this book requires many days of painstaking training and great patience.

Carefully put the above recommendations into practice and you will receive more than enough dividends for your health, physical and mental well-being, as well as an extraordinary state of mind coupled with the feeling of confidence and security that feeling possessed of a wonderful Personal Defense technique provides.

The breathing

In this chapter the reader will learn the most important part of their sports preparation: knowing how to breathe correctly, something that very few people assess in its exact value and that, as we will see later, is essential for the following:

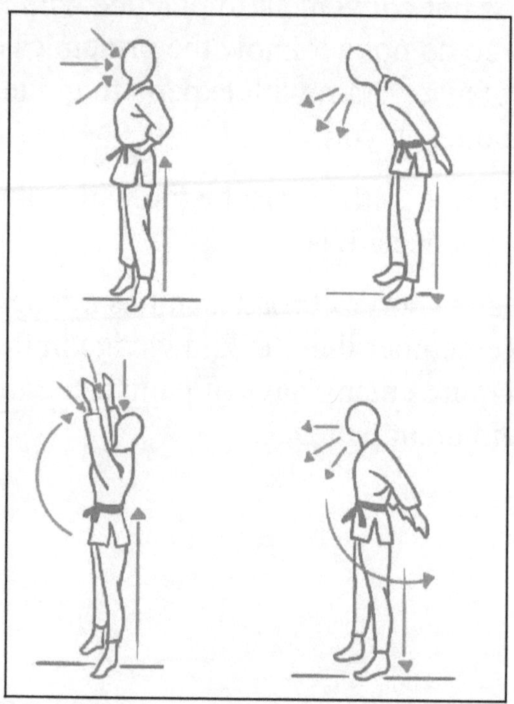

Breathing is living, the most important function of the human body is to breathe because all the others depend on that function. Man will be able to live for some time without eating or drinking, but without breathing, his life would inevitably end in a matter of seconds; This, which is easy to understand, contains the great truth of the success or failure of an athlete, since strong muscles will do him no good, if he does not know how to breathe properly, since the work of the heart and lungs is much more vital than that of muscles; however, this goes unnoticed by many applicants.

The heart and its important functions work outside the control of our will, but through the physical preparation exercises that I describe in the corresponding chapter, the collaboration of this organ can be obtained.

In contrast to the heart, the lungs are capable of being controlled by our will, as long as we strive to achieve it through the intelligent training that I describe below.

From this moment we will begin the study and practice of a good breathing system.

Let us always remember that good breathing translates into a physical and mental state of improvement, since breathing provides man with the necessary oxygen to purify his blood, expelling carbonic acid, influencing blood circulation and intervening in an endless list of bodily benefits.

There are two ways to breathe, which are:

A. The common breath that we all know, which we will call superior.

B. Complete, lower or diaphragmal breathing, which is what we will see in the lines ahead.

The first way of breathing, known worldwide to man, does not need study, since we acquire it from the moment of birth, giving with it the beginning of life; this way of breathing uses the upper part of the lungs.

The complete, lower and diaphragmal breathing is one of the most valuable attributes of Yoga; It is not easy to learn, as it requires constant training, in accordance with the rules indicated below:

Stand at attention, breathe deeply, with all the expansion that you can give to your lungs, in order to fill them to their full capacity with life-giving oxygen; first fill the upper part of them, then the lower one, making the oxygen reach the diaphragm, holding it for about fifteen seconds and then slowly expelling it through the mouth; breathe again, filling the lower part of the lungs with oxygen, putting into play the diaphragm, which, when descending, exerts pressure on the abdominal organs and pushes the front wall of the abdomen filling the middle region of the lungs, making the lower ribs and sternum; then fill the upper part of the lungs, raising the upper part of the chest, slightly contracting the abdomen, with whose movement we will help the lungs to fill up to their full capacity; stay in that position for fifteen seconds, then proceed to forcefully expel the stale air that the stomach and lungs contained; The expulsion of the air must be done through the mouth as strongly as possible, blowing it until it is completely empty. Start a new deep breath, bring oxygen back to your stomach; hold for five seconds and expel normally through the nose.

Now let's begin a new absorption of oxygen slowly but deeply, raising our arms and enjoying that wide breath of fresh air that comes gently, millimeter by millimeter, until the lungs and stomach are filled to their full capacity; To clean them of their own impurities, hold the oxygen for a few seconds and proceed to expel it slowly, until you achieve a total relaxation.

The first reading is not enough to understand the complete mechanism of this lower breathing, that is why it is essential to practice it several times, preferably before a mirror, so that its correct operation can be fully assimilated and understood. The ideal place to practice the previous exercises is a place full of trees, the most convenient hours being the first of the day (See the drawings on the page).

The quantity and duration of these breathing practices should be moderate the first days, they will gradually increase as the aspirant becomes familiar with them; When the above is carried out in an intelligent way, we will have stronger, healthier and more controlled lungs, which will act as a tireless spring, giving us vigor and alleviating the fatigue that comes with the sudden movements of the sport that we are about to learn.

The team

All sports need to be carried out with adequate equipment to facilitate their performance. Hence, in order to practice Karate and the Personal Defense sets that are discussed here, my readers will also need to equip themselves properly; For this I recommend a three-piece outfit consisting of a sturdy jacket or kimono, loose pants, a jockstrap and a band that serves as a belt, made of thick fabric or cotton, sewn with stitching, with strong cotton cord; thin canvas is recommended, stitched with diamond-shaped seams, in order to give it greater resistance; the trousers will be a bit loose to avoid tearing easily and will be adjusted to the waist with braids of the same fabric, placed as the type known as a drawstring;

The feet will be barefoot if possible, with the nails well trimmed; If necessary, they can be put on with glove-type shoes used by apparatus gymnasts or parkour shoes, and in the latter case, tennis shoes with laces, without metal terminals, can be used only in special cases, since the sport must be practiced barefoot ; Keep fingernails as trimmed as possible and do not wear any kind of rings.

It is necessary to acquire a training bag, like the one boxers use for their practices, a table to practice the chop (I will detail this in subsequent chapters) and a container that can be a bucket full of lentils, or wood shavings for train the hand. Once you have the elements indicated above, we will be able to start our sports activities.

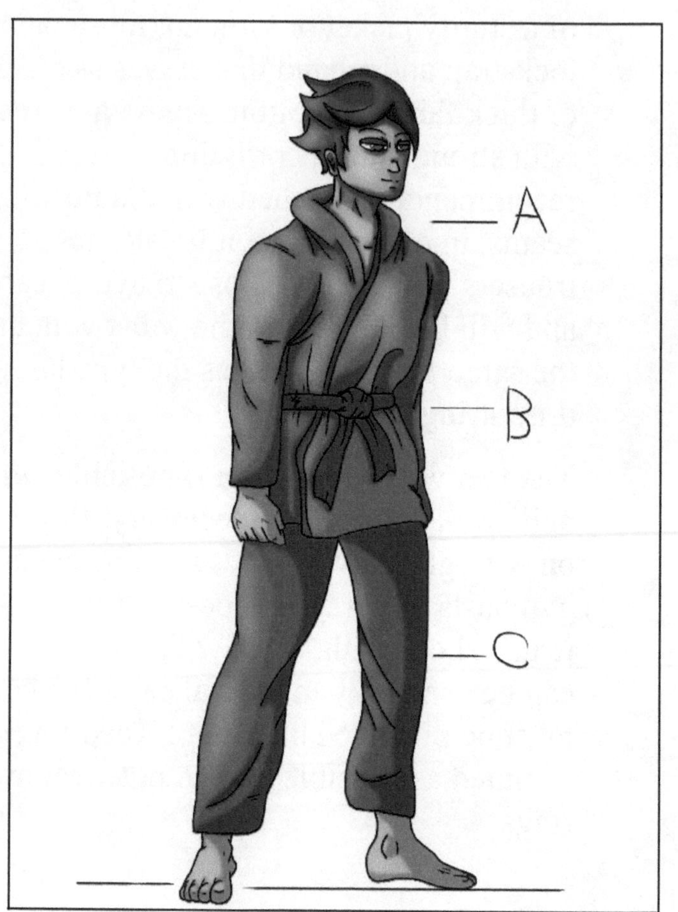

Where and how to practice this sport

After the previous training to find the necessary physical condition in order to enter fully into the practice of skirmishes, the aspirant will find himself full of vitality, his muscles will have been hardened and his mind will be ready to take action.

For this, we need a suitable place to test the theory of this treatise and convert what is presented in block letters into positive results; the ideal place should be a clean, well-ventilated place, without noises, equipped with a dojo, that is, a mattress of approximately four meters per side that will be placed on a wooden platform; The mattress must be filled with soft materials and lined with a resistant canvas such as those used in the ring where Olympic wrestling is practiced, neither too hard that does not protect the body from the roughness of falls, nor too soft that allows the feet sink, as this would lead to the consequent loss of speed; in case of not being able to count on such a mattress, the workouts can be done outdoors, on the grass.

Once the site has been decided where the essential elements mentioned are to be found, the skirmishes could begin, having to practice these with a partner of the same age, size and weight, being necessary that the first sets be jealously watched by an expert, or at least by someone initiated in the matter, who will have the mission of helping the correct execution of the sets and who must also correct the defects of the applicants, in order to avoid the creation of vices, and ensure the physical safety of the initiates, leading them by the hand, as it were, in their pininos within this sport, in which the primary phase is the most important to care for.

When the aspirants have successfully passed this first aspect and begin to show skillfulness, then the practice will alternate with stronger men, of different heights and weights, who gradually will physically and mentally blanket the aspirant, affirming with this and with each new practice their knowledge. In the event that the third man I refer to as a watchdog cannot be counted on, I recommend that the practice be carried out with great prudence, marking only, not throwing yourself deeply in the execution of the casts. To avoid counterproductive results, this process of marking and not pulling will slow down learning, but will definitely be safer; when a set is well understood, execute it completely,

Hygiene Rules

Every athlete requires both a zealous care of their behavior, and a strict observance of hygiene rules, in order to achieve the ideal state of health that allows their improvement in sport.

In order to achieve the above, below, I insert ten rules of conduct, of rigid sports discipline, that will beneficially increase your health, physical and mental well-being.

I.   Get up early, perform breathing exercises, gymnastics and a light training of the topics discussed here.

II.   Sleeping a minimum of eight hours a day on average, or naps of six hours.

III.   Get away from vices and excesses.

IV.   Eat well, at the right time, abundant vegetables, red meat, fish, little flour and fat.

V.   Tone up with vitamins of natural or herbal origin moderately.

VI.   Many sun baths and walks in the open air.

VII.   Monitoring your weight and your health.

VIII.   Scrupulous observance of cleanliness and hygiene.

IX.   Periodic medical check-ups.

X.   Strict sports discipline, so as not to miss a single day without training and without stopping to carry out the aforementioned rules.

XI.   Periodic medical check-ups.

XII.   Strict sports discipline, so as not to miss a single day without training and without stopping to carry out the rules noted above.

By carrying out what has been stated in previous lines, the applicant will obtain as a reward for his perseverance the greatest treasure that exists under the sun and that is health; therefore, let us always remember this wise sentence:

- **God always forgives ...**

- **Man sometimes ...**

- **Nature never ...**

Let us take care with the greatest possible zeal that precious gift with which nature has endowed us: Health.

Learning to spring

It is understood by spring or sprung movements, all those made with great speed and vigor, tending to facilitate a lightning attack or a fast exit.

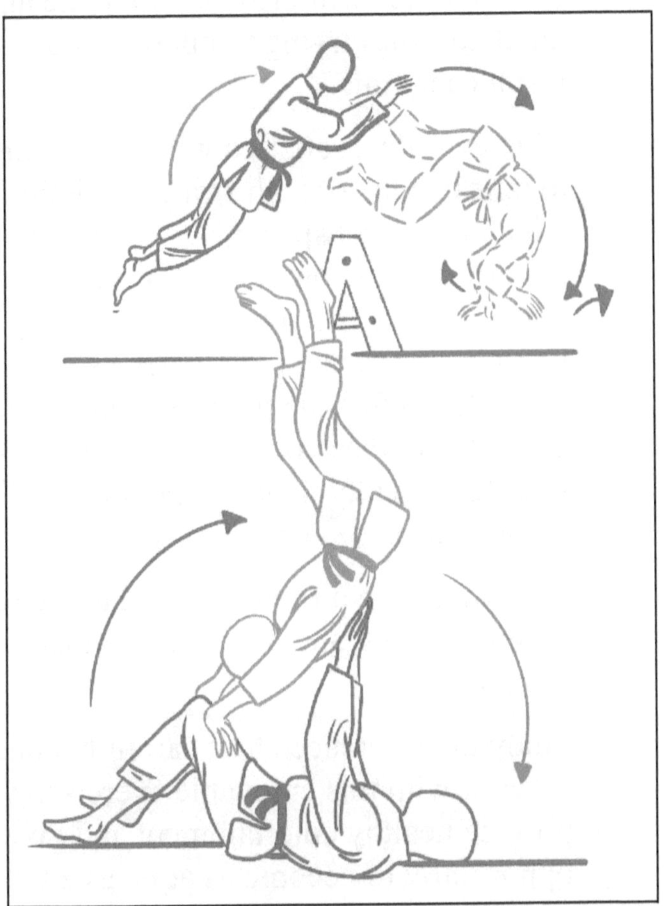

The main springs are in the thighs and waist, but all our muscles are susceptible to spring, if we have previously prepared them for it.

In the previous graph, the springs and their most common preparation exercises are illustrated; the "A" presents the one derived from the exercise known as the squat, from which a jump that provides feline agility comes out; perform the aforementioned squat exercise, and when jumping try to get the most out of the spring that your muscles will provide; do it one and a hundred times trying to obtain a more spirited result each time.

When you feel satisfied with that spring, go on to rehearse the one illustrated with the letter "B", which is a waist spring, very simple to execute; to perform it lie on your back with your back flat to the ground, lift your legs vigorously with a waist spring, make them reach as high as possible, so that the point of support on the ground becomes your lungs; in the air spring your feet vividly towards the four cardinal points, this based on a spring.

Let's finish the aforementioned exercise by giving a strong and quick spring that makes us stand up.

Study the reference chart carefully and proceed to work with this enjoyable exercise, which will provide healthy entertainment and give you the opportunity to become as agile as a bobcat.

Now we will go on to practice a very easy spring. To do this, study figure "D" in the illustrated graph, in which there is a movement tending to bring the palms of the hands to the ground; To facilitate the above, make a spring by forcing the waist back, which, when returning to the front and down, will do so in a natural way, with great simplicity and making it easier to touch the ground with the palms of the hands.

With the previous examples and with springs of his own inventiveness, the reader should expand his repertoire of springs every day, which will be very useful when we get into the practice of the skirmishes that I will present in the next chapters.

I recommend practicing the exercise known as "tiger jump" that is illustrated in the graph, due to the excellent results it reports.

Preparation of the hands

In this chapter we will deal with a basic theme for the sport that concerns us in this treatise and that is to gradually harden the hands until they become strong blacksmith's pliers; To achieve this, the exercises illustrated in the graph must be practiced daily, which consist of:

A. Open and close the hand vigorously, not less than one hundred times in each series.

B. Squeeze a sponge ball with your fingertips.

C. Execute movements from front to back of the fist.

D. Lift a chair or similar object, using pressure with the fingers, without arching the wrist or arm.

E. Rotation exercises of the hand with the fist tightly closed, towards the four cardinal points, alternating movements. To relax the muscles from the previous exercises, loosen your fingers and shake your hands vigorously, whipping your fingers, which will give you immediate relief; Consistency in the daily practice of these exercises, after a few months the reader will have strong hands, agile and sturdy fingers and a solid wrist, with which we will have barely climbed the first step of the series that will lead him to be a good karate performer.

Do not rush and want in a short time to achieve what normally requires many years of preparation, remember that your hands are going to be the working tools in this virile sport, in which only those who demonstrate tenacity stand out.

Therefore, willingly submit to the foregoing practices; be your own trainer, increase the amount and time of the exercises, as is convenient and your muscles respond to you in the same way; do not go overboard, but do not do less than you consider necessary; always maintain the same upward rhythm of work.

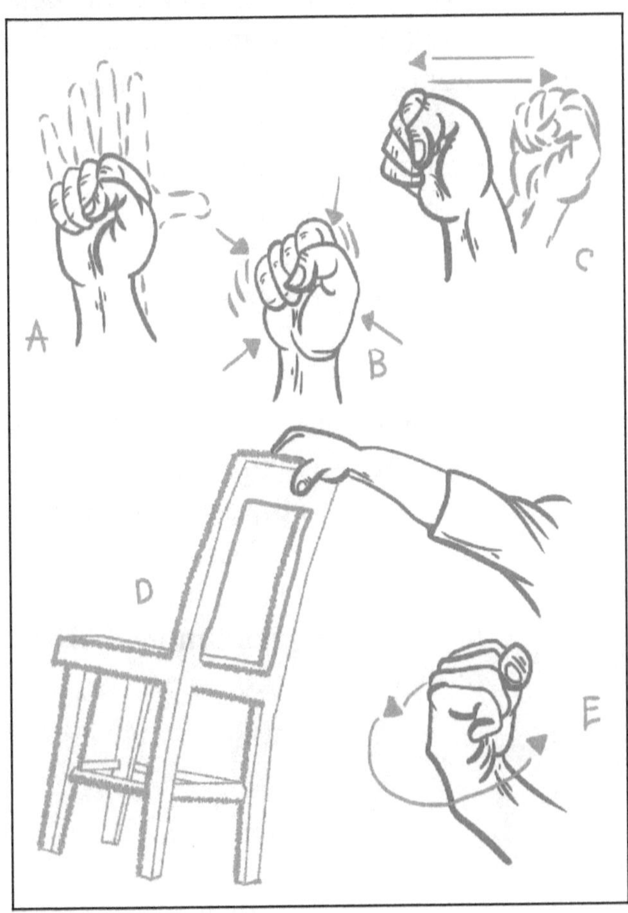

The Tagus

When the reader's hands are sufficiently hardened with the exercises in the previous chapter, he will be able to start practicing this devastating blow, which appears to be easy but requires a long time of training to make it effective and forceful; for your practice get a board approximately fifty centimeters long by twenty wide and three centimeters thick, place it on your thighs and practice the strike by stopping the plank with the left hand while striking with the right and vice versa; This daily practice should be done by striking a minimum of one hundred times with each hand, increasing or decreasing the power of the blow, as the hand supports the impacts.

We will start with more or less strong cuts, interspersing soft blows to rest, giving blows from time to time with maximum power; these at first will occur less frequently; time will get us used to more solid impacts since the edge of the hand this day with more resistant day and the blow is more accurate.

Practice the cut on a sack like the one used by boxers or with the lined board of the Kataristas, hitting in different places, sending the cut from different starting angles. To master this shot from all imaginable starting points and that it comes out well, accurately and hard from all of them, I recommend not getting delighted the first few times by hitting too hard, as it may hurt your hand; Mastery of the pit is obtained after one year of daily practice.

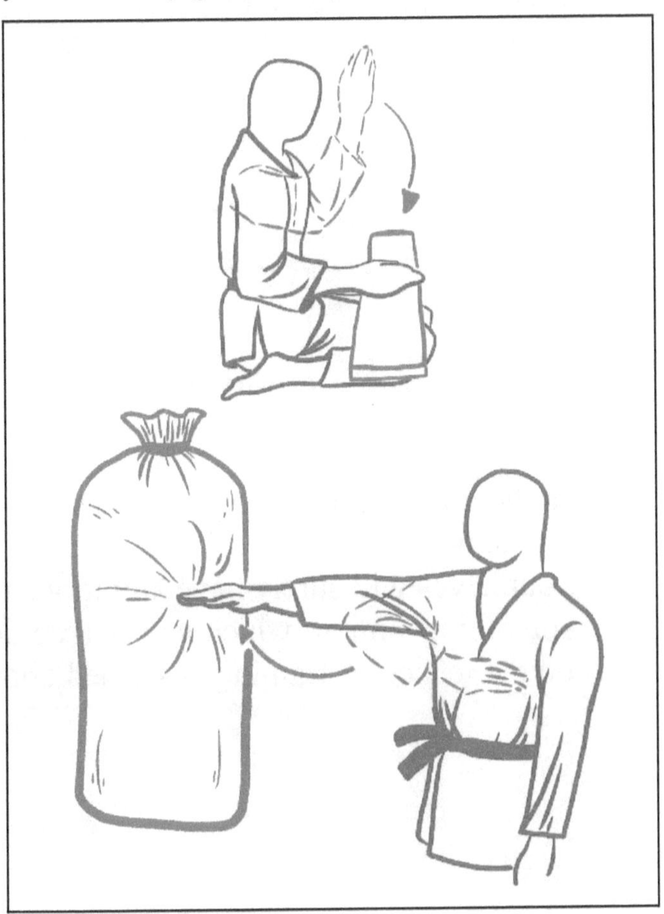

In my sporting life I have met more than a dozen karate performers who, after more than twenty years of daily training this blow, managed to break a brick one inch thick with relative ease; These extraordinary displays are only possible, as I previously noted, after many years of constant work, hence my recommendation to readers to arm themselves with a lot of patience and tirelessly practice this wonderful knowledge, which will surely pay you handsomely for the time you dedicate to it.

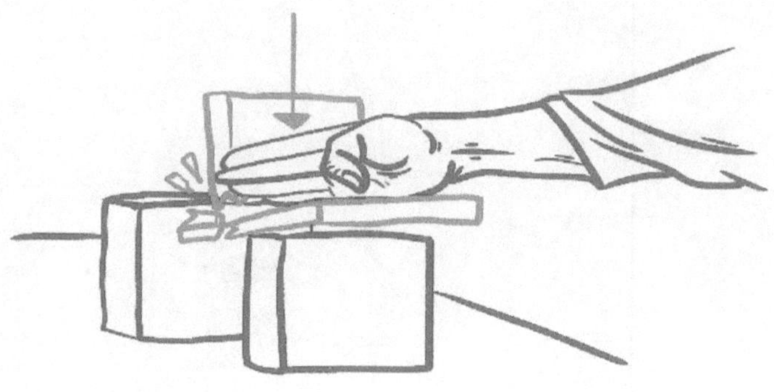

In the drawing of the graph, a master block stroke is illustrated, breaking a board; You yourselves will surely have ambitions to do something similar, which you will achieve based on the tenacious training described above.

WARNING

The knowledge that the reader will see in the following chapters is extremely rough and dangerous; For this reason, I recommend a lot of prudence and chivalry during your training sessions.

Karate weapons

As we have previously established, the word Karate means "empty hand" or hand without weapons. However, the true technique of this sport has turned the hands, elbows, fingers, knees and feet into powerful combat weapons, thanks to special training.

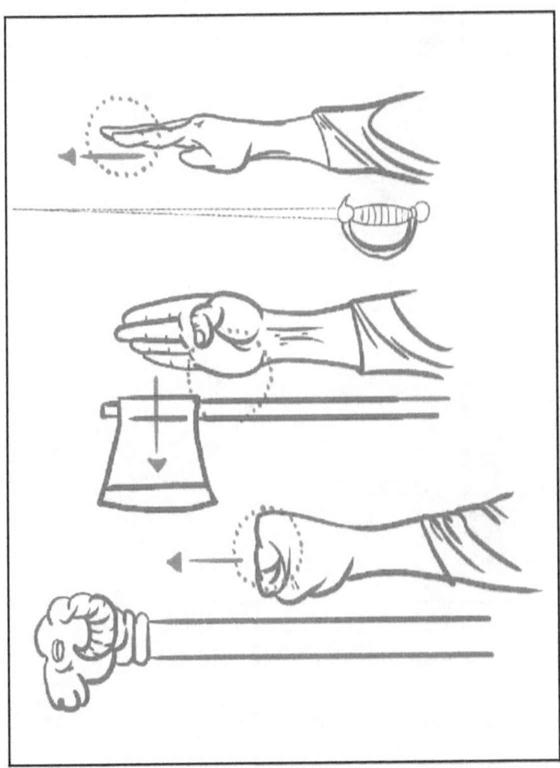

In the following graphs, our natural weapons are illustrated; next to them are a series of drawings that symbolically show the forceful kind of combat element they become; Having control over these weapons is not easy, it requires adequate physical conditioning, so that they can offer the returns of several years, in order to have them well organized in our favor.

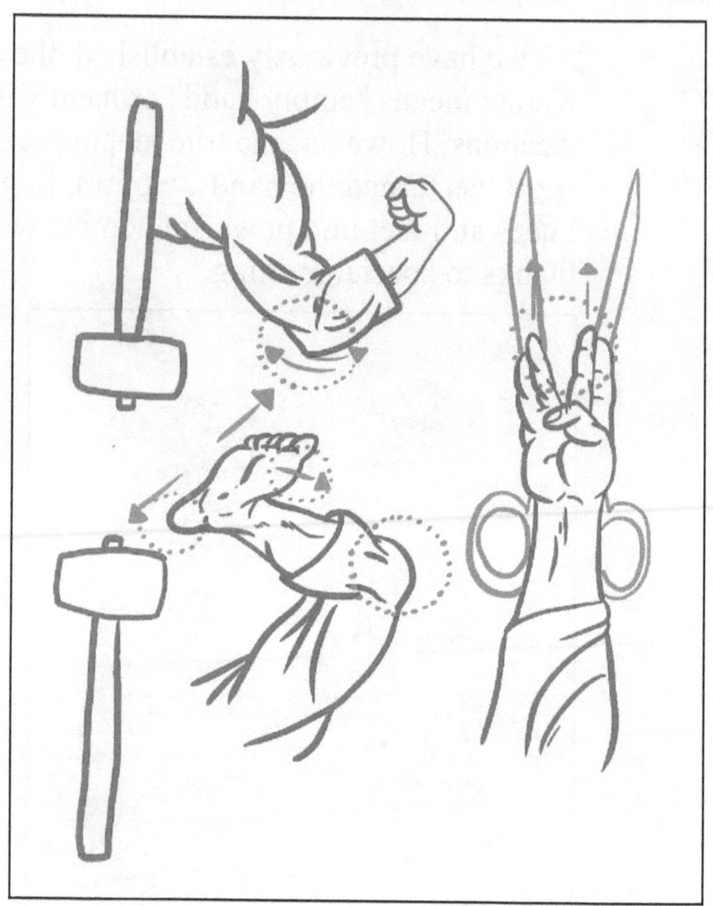

The reader should be made, from that moment, to the idea of studying and practicing a lot and for many years, in order to crystallize the desire that led him to buy this book, which is to become possessor of wonderful knowledge, the Which will provide both the way to defend himself scientifically from any physical attack, as well as to be a strong man, healthy in body and mind, owner of a strong body, with quick reflexes, strong muscles and great agility.

But all this, I insist, will only be obtained after long hours of rough and intense training, with many hours of the gym stolen from our activities, a complete abstention from all kinds of human vices and weaknesses.

Since the Karate performer requires zealous observance of rules of conduct, not only physical but also mental.

So, let's study the reference drawings carefully to understand the message of their symbols and, without further ado, let's start the steps that will allow us to turn them into virtuous performers of this virile sport.

Vulnerable parts of the body

The drawings in this graph indicate which are the vulnerable points of the body, in order to harden those that are susceptible to it.

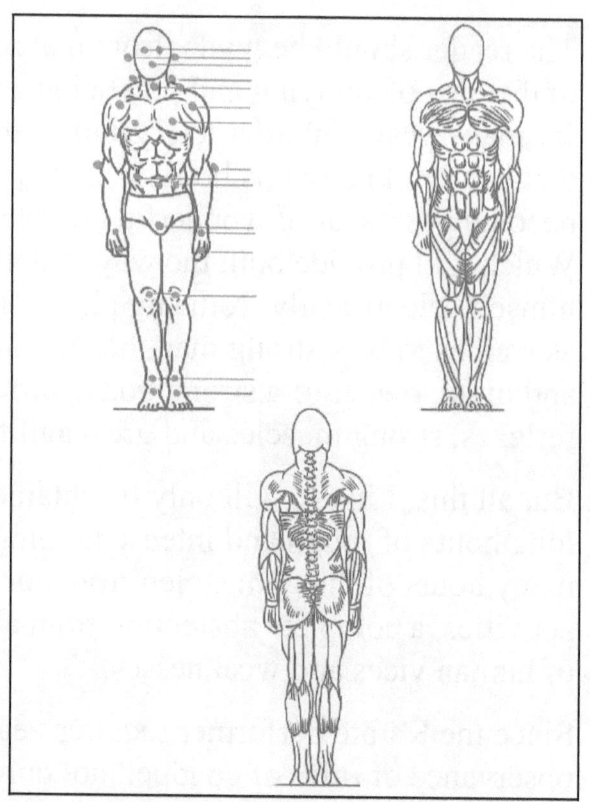

Karate punch with the base of the palm of the hand

In the illustrations of the graphics present, there are drawings that show another of the wonderful resources of that amazing range that Karate offers; In it, the base of the palm of the hand is used to hit and deflect blows, block both kicks and blows with the fist or slash, aimed at places identified as vulnerable. To use this resource it is necessary to learn to present the hand properly, in order to avoid injuring the fingers; either hand is used interchangeably.

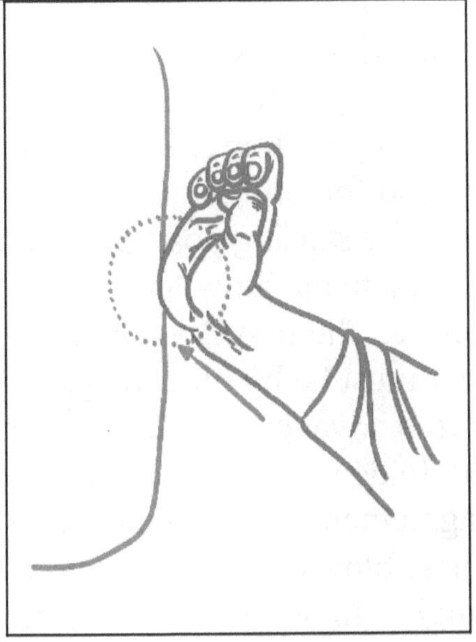

To get into the subject, carefully study the illustrations inserted in the lines above; prepare your hand and let's start with the shadow exercise performed in front of a mirror, looking for the ideal style for its execution; When you have achieved this first aspect, we will proceed to the practice of formal striking against the sack, in order to harden the hand and the roughness of its impacts; Of course, this blow should not be changed in any case to one that we can apply with a closed fist, this is elementary logic, but we must recognize the efficiency of this throw when fighting short we can hit hard with this blow the lower part of the base of the opponent's nose, to which we will materially pulverize it; Thus,

In the blocking plan, it should be practiced deflecting marking strokes that both in learning and in blank, the practice partner will send us; Try to make all your impacts extraordinarily fast, strong and forceful, immediately returning your hand to the starting position, that is, on guard; accentuate the blow harshly to make it more effective; The first days of practice with your partner must be by mutual agreement, that is, knowing in advance the blow that is going to be blocked, to do so; as its malice increases, the previous agreement will disappear and in its place surprise blows will be thrown from all possible angles, in order to become more decisive and take full advantage of the resources it assimilates.

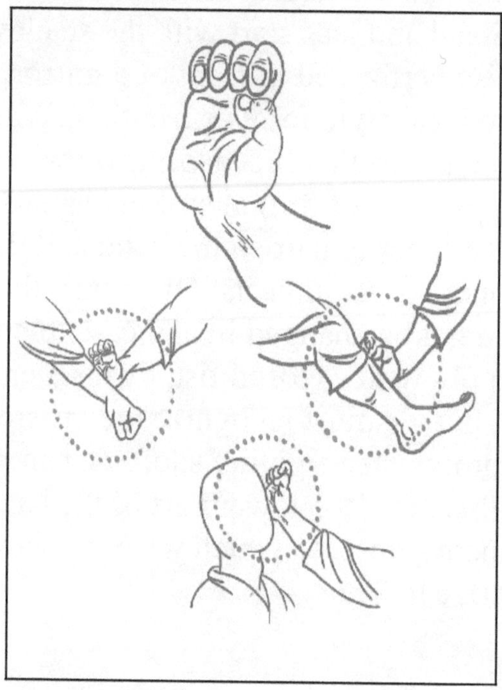

Alternate practicing this strike with both hands to make it more complete; Practice it thoroughly until you feel confident that you know it perfectly and execute it neatly in whatever position you are in.

Karate kick

Now we will study one of the most colorful, spectacular and forceful blows of Karate, which is tipped with the edge of the sole of the foot.

Apart from being very striking, it is used in open fighting, as a self-defense or blocking resource, preparing the ground for more definitive blows and as a softening method, or as a direct attack.

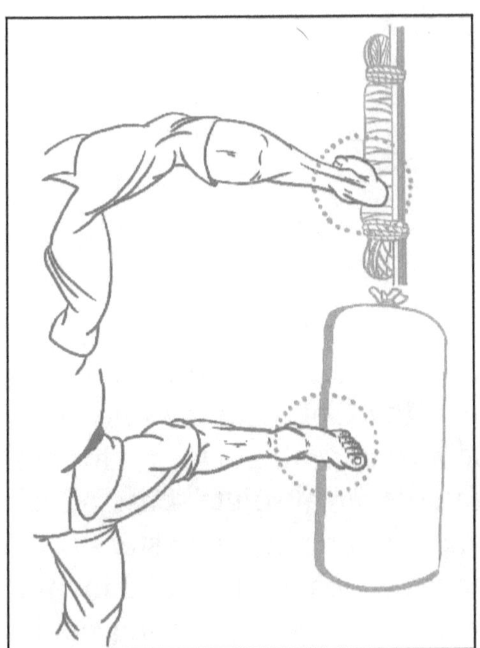

Therefore, it can be appreciated that it is a very broad resource, therefore it is necessary to learn it perfectly.

This blow will be practiced barefoot, necessarily requiring the mirror, since that is where the primary movements are tuned and the execution errors are self-corrected.

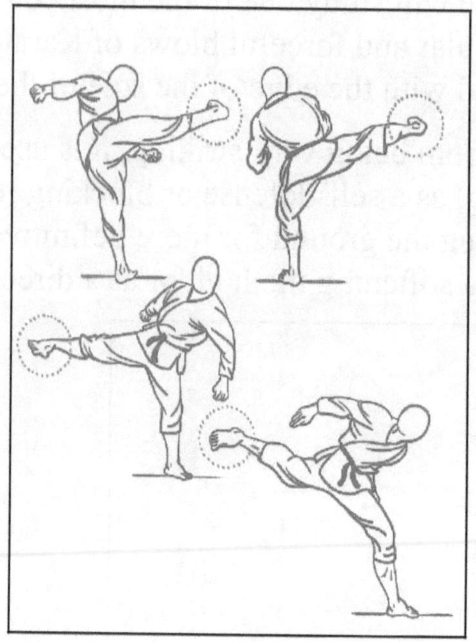

The blow can be delivered with the outer edge of the sole of the foot, with the sole of the foot, with the heel or with the toes. This cast requires a lot of verve, an absolute sense of balance, speed and toughness; To master this blow, patience is needed, months and months of constant and endless mirror and shadow practices, until we achieve the necessary ease and with it begin to practice against the sack or the Makiwara.

It is not advisable to train against the aforementioned elements without first having fluency and agility, since what would be achieved would be counterproductive, that is, a perhaps strong blow, but without any mobility, and the basis of success in this cast is feline agility , coupled with a strong punch of effective aim.

A preliminary exercise to these workouts and that I recommend as ideal, is to jump the rope for a few minutes a day to give your legs some ease.

After the previous recommendations, let's get into the matter by carefully studying the illustrations of the graphs shown, in which the basic movements necessary to achieve effectiveness with this blow are illustrated.

As can be seen, there are two basic aspects: first, standing solidly on one leg, jealously guarding the balance during the fraction of seconds that it remains in the air; second, to get the kick accurately to the desired location.

But they are not crazy or drowning kicks that are thrown, they are scientifically calculated kicks, with calm aim and straight force, so that, when making an impact in the chosen place, the planned dividends are obtained in advance.

When the reader has the necessary agility, ease and speed ideal for this blow, then, not before, we will formally train him against the sack, in order to obtain the punch that gives the impact against something resistant; To do this, let's study the graph, which illustrates a hitting training against a sack or Makiwara.

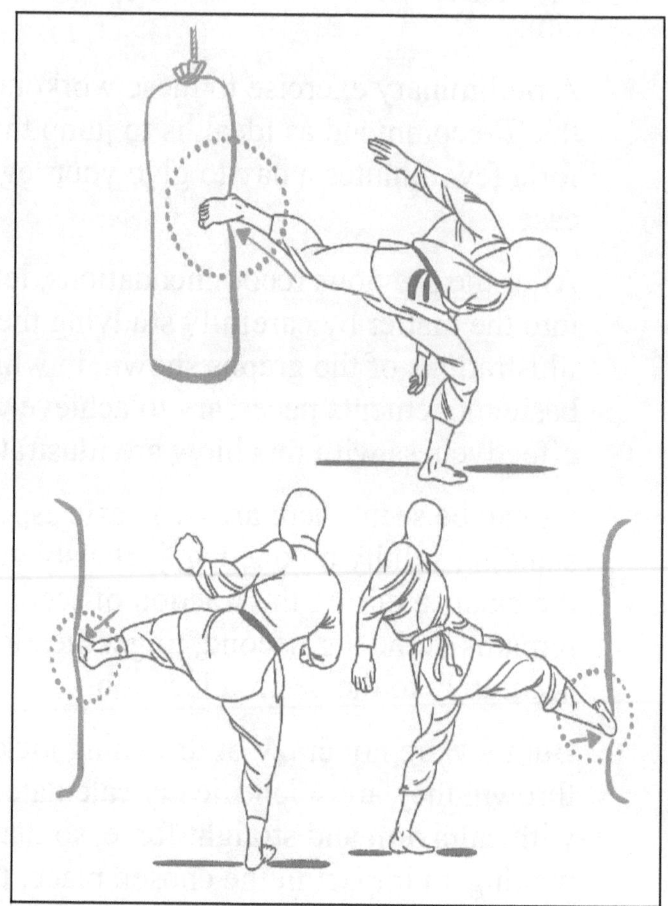

I leave this accessory to your choice, but my recommendation is to start the first practices with great measure, taking care that the blow is the most classic and well executed, without worrying about the moment that it is strong, since the most important thing in the first phase, is to take care of the correct execution, watching the figure, the balance; the hit will come with time, as you acquire form, security and confidence in your style and toughness.

We will observe in the aforementioned graph, that the blow is applied indistinctly with either of the two legs, that the impact is achieved by striking with the edge of the outer side of the sole of the foot, which is the one that produces a more painful blow; When making contact with the sack, the foot should be slightly arched to strike precisely at the designated spot; When this blow is well digested, we will go on to study it, but applying it with the heel; This launch will already be easier for our readers, but anyway much work will have to be done with it to achieve the required accuracy.

When you consider that you have learned this blow well, we will go on to practice it, but making contact with the base of the toes, being necessary to take great care of its correct execution so as not to hurt yourself.

With the above, we will end this cast in terms of applying it barefoot. With shoes it is also used by expanding its radius of action by hitting with the toe and the edge of the sole, which covers the inside of the foot. In later chapters we will review their breadth.

To finish, I want to state that this blow must be combined with a chain of subsequent blows that completes a complete and devastating attack.

Remember the reader that perseverance and long hours of training will be the only thing that will give you the possession of this extraordinary resource, which I consider the most important of Karate sets.

Karate Knee Strike

Within the resources of Karate, there is the blow that is applied with the knee, which, like all of this sport, is extremely dangerous; It takes a lot of toughness and a conscientious between birth to be able to turn it into something truly useful as an element of defense and attack.

Well, getting into the subject, let's proceed to study the graph in which the set of this chapter is illustrated.

The knee is lavished, precisely, with the edge of the knee and is always directed to eminently vulnerable places; both knees can be used.

The coup itself is quite simple, its execution rudimentary; In reality, great classicism is not required, but a source of speed, elasticity, strength and aim is required, to always hit the previously set target, this of course without telegraphing movements that put the opponent on guard; This part is fundamental, since the knee should be a surprising and devious blow.

His training is against the sack or Makiwara, and, as in all cases, we will begin to practice it in front of the mirror, in order to understand his exact trajectory, the height that can be reached, as well as his distance to have the blow measured and always send it with the assurance that it will hit the target.

This blow is used in hand-to-hand fights, in the field that in boxing is known as "fighting short"; My recommendation for the success of this cast is to prepare it with shadow exercises, vigorously raising the knee, taking care that the weight of your body is well balanced on the other leg, so as not to lose even one iota of balance, since if this happened , the launch would be counterproductive; Therefore, let us watch this vital aspect in our shadow exercises, which will be further rounded when it is executed in front of the mirror in which we can be our own judges, and see if we leave a possible gap through which the opposite can filter, or if our bad or inadequate position is conducive for them to work against us.

To avoid the above, I suggest doing the following: Appearing to rest firmly on the soles of your feet, bend your knees slightly forward and raise them as high as you can.

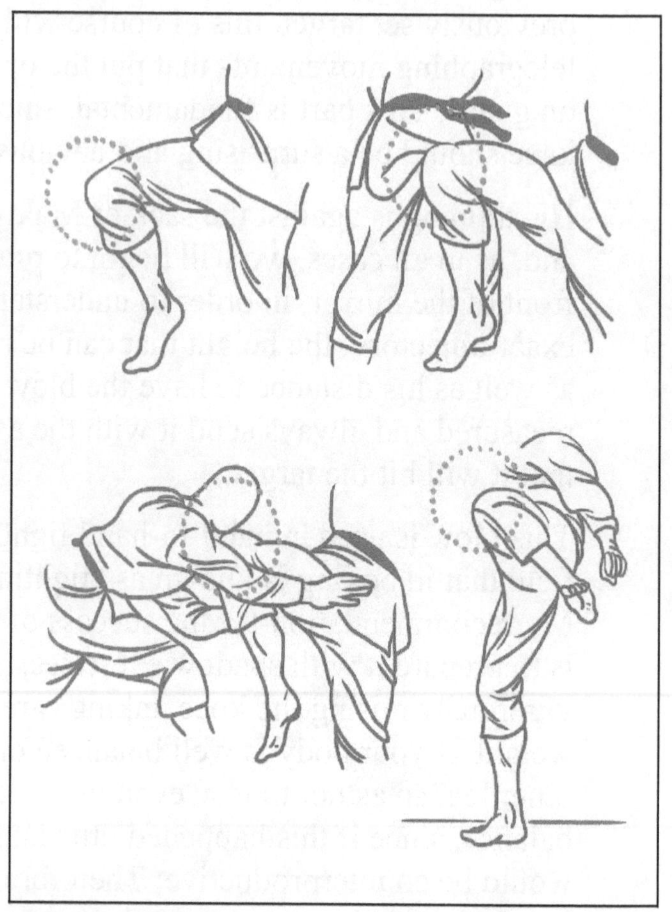

The second exercise consists of throwing the knee as far forward as possible. Combining these exercises, we will measure our target distance.

After these preliminaries, we will go on to train the blow against the sack, trying to gain strength, but without neglecting the aim, returning it in fractions of a second to its starting point, to stay on guard with perfectly controlled balance.

Karate blows with the hand

Karate has an extensive repertoire of blows that are applied with the hand, using various positions of these. The following graphic illustrates five different ways of hitting with the hand, let's study each drawing carefully to perfectly capture how to use each of these extraordinary resources correctly.

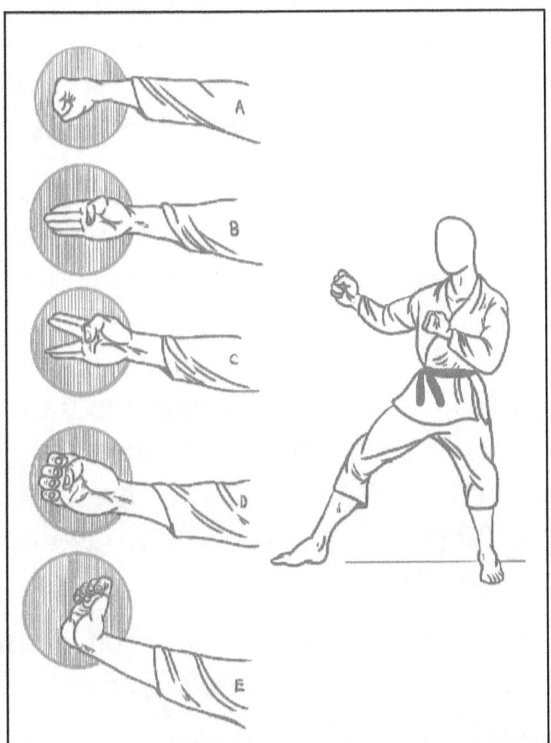

Figure "A" shows the closed fist, a blow known to all as Boxing, but in Karate this blow comes out of the guard position that appears in the drawing of the complete doll, achieves its impact by making a corkscrew movement that gives a strong impulse to the blow, which is forceful and devastating.

In due course we will detail both the correct form of your training and the means of obtaining greater dividends from it.

Figure "B" shows the hand in a position to attack striking with the tips of the fingers; To use this blow, it is necessary to conscientiously harden hands and fingers with a series of special trainings that we will see in later chapters; This blow will always be directed to soft, vulnerable parts; When this coup is well established, its results are radical.

The figure that appears marked with the letter "C", presents another way of using the fingers, presenting them in a V shape as indicated. For the layman, opening the fingers in this position is difficult since it is necessary to train this movement many times to achieve the necessary ease and to do it as a reflex; This blow is dangerous, as it is always aimed at the opponent's eyes.

It cannot and should not be practiced in the gym, at the most shading, knowing exactly where it will end up, but that's it.

When you use this resource, it will be because your life is in danger, as it is one of the secret blows of Karate, perhaps the most bloody, for which I recommend to my readers extreme caution in its practice and subsequent use.

I insist, it will only be used in extreme cases. Talk about the position of "Clenched Fist": Open your hand quickly in such a way that when you open it, your fingers are in the said V position; do it hundreds of times until it is run smoothly.

The figure indicated by the letter "D" shows a hand with a semi-closed fist; the blow on this occasion is carried out by the knuckles of the second joint of the fingers; study exactly the place with which the impact will be applied, once assimilated in theory, we will get to know it in practice.

This resource is another strong blow that occurs in weak parts, with devastating results.

Of course, you have to know the places where the greatest impact is achieved and the ideal way to obtain better results; As with the aforementioned resource, care must be taken in its practice and only used in cases where it is truly indispensable.

Finally, we have the illustration marked with the letter "E".

In it the way of striking with the base of the palm of the hand is presented; This knowledge is extraordinary, not only for attack, but for blocking and defense, being its way of applying easy to understand; This blow will always be directed to previously known places, where its impact is definitive or to avoid, blocking, the opponent's blows.

Let's go back again to the figure of the letter "B", which I intentionally left the last to make the reader notice that from this position of the hand comes the blow known by the Tagus, which I detail in full detail in a special chapter; This stroke complements the series of resources for striking with the hand.

Now, after having known in theory these radical knowledge of attack and self-defense, we will go on to train them properly so that they become natural reflexes, and that they can be used as easily as an experienced driver changes the speeds of his car; For this we must first toughen the hand, fingers and wrists; then learn to place the fingers in the indicated positions, doing it quickly as normal movement of the same.

In the chapter on preparing the hands, I fully explain the special exercises aimed at preparing your hands for these rough hitting training that we need to get the hands and fingers to respond appropriately; don't try to skip the preparation off your hands, it would be counterproductive.

There are people who by birth have strong hands, but their strength is not adequate for these impacts, therefore, all my readers should without excuse or pretext, train properly before entering fully into the practice of this knowledge.

Karate punches with the elbow

In real karate the elbows are also used to strike; Therefore, today I will introduce my readers to the knowledge of a new resource, in which, as previously noted, elbows are used; This blow is very forceful, it carries the weight of the one who gives it and its results are like all Karate blows, devastating.

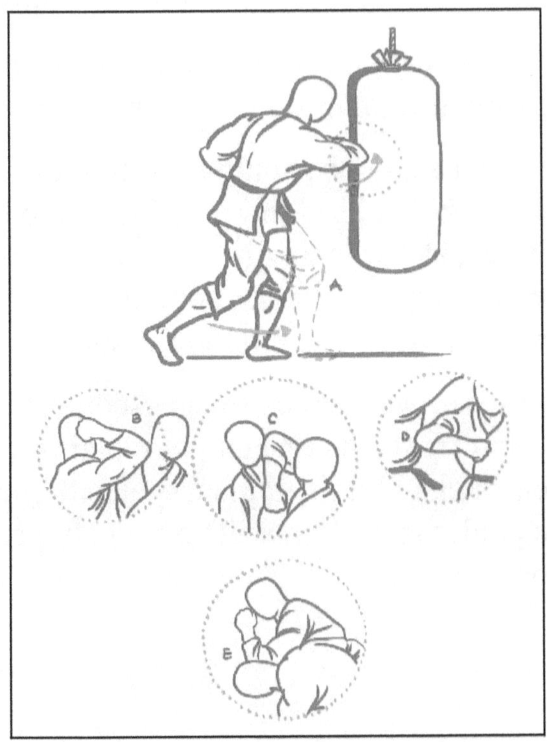

In the illustrations of the graph there are drawings of some of its forms of application and training; Let's study them carefully and put into practice.

The classic training of Karate blows is done against a Makiwara, which is a board lined with soft, firm and sturdy materials, but I advise departing somewhat from this classicism and training against a sack like those used by boxers during their practices. Since it has the advantage over the Makiwara, it is completely passive.

But, finally, if this seems better to the reader, you can use it; its well-known purpose is to harden, get aim, punch and perfect movements.

So either with the sack or the Makiwara, let's start the formal hitting training.

The first sessions should be extremely light, without being used thoroughly, to avoid possible injuries; as hardening is achieved, the power of the blows will increase, not before; remember that in the slow assimilation is success.

The strike with the elbow is used in short, close combat fights; its impact goes against previously identified and trained places; Needless to say, the reader is dealing with extremely painful blows.

For your formal training, stand in front of the sack at the distance your elbow needs to make contact, and you must be perfectly standing, balancing your body weight so as not to lose even one iota of balance; When striking, help give it greater force with the waist spring, bearing the weight of the body and carrying it with the elbow; upon impact, it will immediately return to its starting place.

Don't gobble up when hitting and lose balance or distance; Practice the impact of the elbow starting from different angles of departure, either placing the fist upwards in a horizontal or diagonal position, pointing the fist downwards, always looking for better aim and greater consistency.

To be effective, we must practice daily fine-tuning details, without overlooking the slightest.

Karate punch with the fist

In Karate there is a blow that is delivered with a closed fist, let's say equal to the blows of Boxing, unlike ours has more forceful effects; For it, the fist of the hand is used with the fingers perfectly closed, topped by the thumb, which goes over the index and middle fingers, for greater consistency.

Look carefully at the correct way to close the hand, which is illustrated in the following graphic, and let's move on to the training of this blow, which, according to the canons of Karate, should be practiced against a Makiwara, but I have modernized this aspect by recommending the use of a boxing training bag. Well, in one place or another, the fundamental thing is to practice it exhaustively until it is perfectly done.

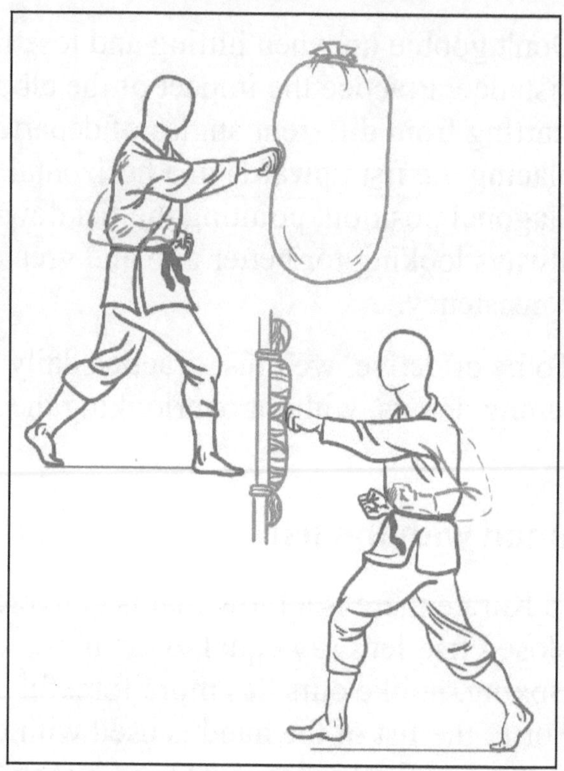

For your understanding, let's study the graph in which two figures appear training said blow, in one the sack is seen, in the other the blow is against a Makiwara; This is a thick board solidly secured to the floor, lined in the part where you train, with material that can be henequen or a similar fiber, then lined with adhesive fabric bandages to give it body.

Returning to the point that interests us, the blow comes out of the guard position, that is, at the height of his belt, the hand with his thumb pointed upwards; to strike the fist is brought forward, making a corkscrew movement, so that upon reaching its destination and making contact, the fist is turned downward, pointing the thumb to the ground; This corkscrew movement is essential, because that is precisely where the point of the blow is located.

To fix the exact placement and travel of the arm, first train in front of a mirror, and when this blow goes well, proceed to perform it against the sack making contact, seeking that each time the blow is stronger, taking good care of the first days; In order not to injure your hands, it is advisable to bandage them following the technique used by boxers. The legs should be solidly seated on the ground, so that the impact is more solid and safe.

With the previous practice, the hands become too hard and they lose ability for manual work; hence, if the reader works with them in their normal activities, they should take care not to atrophy them with the practices I have been referring to.

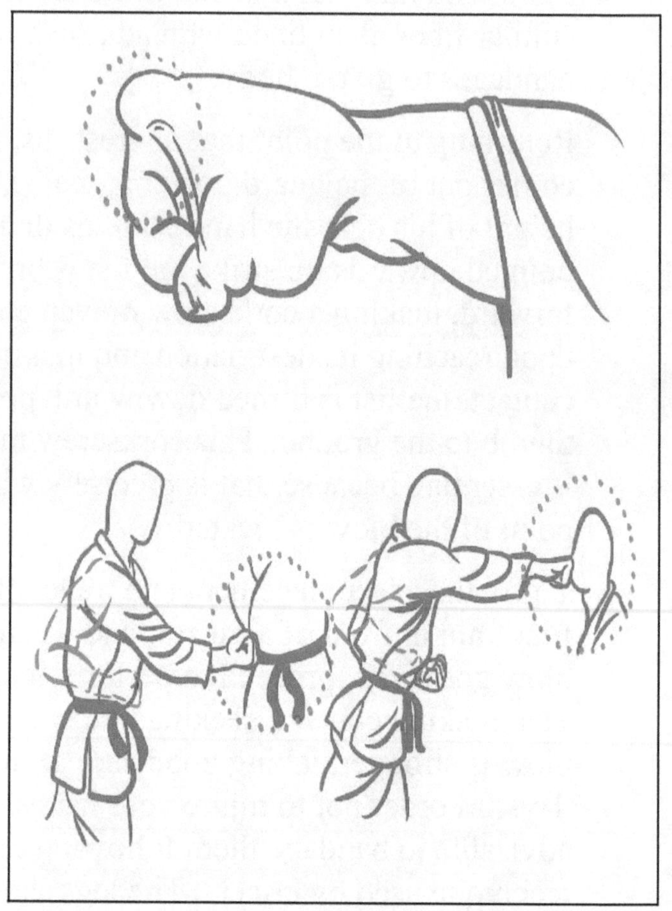

After each session of approximately fifty strokes per hand against the sack, do the training in shadow, without enemy in front, correcting the figure, to make your movements cleaner and more elegant.

For a better understanding, we will detail the rules, which are: first, placement of the legs in front of the sack, solidly seated on the floor, knees slightly bent to draw spring from the thighs, the waist as loose as possible, in order to obtain spring from her and take the hit more quickly; the weight of the body should be let go intelligently in each stroke to give it forceful power, but taking care not to lose balance; a katarista must be an expert in not leaving like a fighting bull.

The head must have the chin tucked in, pressing it against the chest so as not to offer it as a target; the men loose, the fist tightly closed, but not too tight so as not to tire.

Closing the fist tightly tightens the muscles, hindering agility, weakening the power of the blow.

These details appear to be insignificant, but they are of capital importance, for which we must carefully monitor them so as not to fall into vices that could adversely affect later practices.

Now let's remember the corkscrew movement, which, I insist, must be perfect for us. To do this, we return to the mirror and in slow motion we will carefully observe how this turn is made; this spinal movement must be carefully worked out.

To rest the hand from blows, the reader executes the shadow exercises illustrated in the graph, which loosen the tension and serve to create the block to blows of this type; I recommend my readers to study my book on boxing, since in it the various forms of blocking boxing blows are explained in detail, this will help them to better understand the blocking technique; for now we will focus on marking exercises with a partner, blocking the blows to which we have been referring, stopping them with a closed fist or deflecting them with an outward and downward slash; This training must be done by mutual agreement, on the basis of only marking the blows without impact, since this would result in mutually injuring each other, and what we are trying to do is learn; therefore practice with utmost care,

When releasing the blow, aim at the place where you want to hit the target and make sure that it reaches it exactly.

This is the objective of the intense practice to which they must undergo.

Slash with the foot

In this chapter I will present another interesting Judo resource: using the foot as a cut, to knock down, protect or attack.

In the graph, the exact place of the foot that is used to apply the cut is illustrated, presenting its form of training.

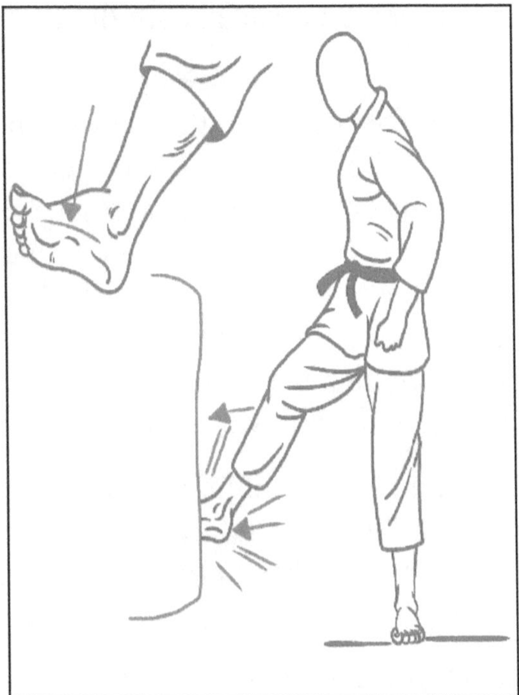

In order to achieve absolute mastery over this resource, we need a long practice similar to that used to train the cut with the hand.

Therefore, the applicant must resign himself to working for a minimum of one year to be able to learn the exact application of the cut with the foot.

The first thing to do is to try to strengthen the foot and ankle by doing the following exercise: standing at attention, lift your body on the balls of your feet, balancing it in that place; do this exercise a minimum of fifty times daily.

Then we will practice the blow against a sack like the one boxers use in their training sessions, taking the first blows wearing tennis shoes, in order to prepare and accustom the foot to impacts.

When you feel strong in this regard, then the training will be barefoot; The correct way to apply this blow is, at the same time, fast, accurate, forceful and continued with a strong push, in which all the weight of the body will be carried to move the practice bag, so that when it is applied against the companion, it is easily knocked down whatever his weight or height.

As indicated in the graph, the sack should be struck with one foot and maintaining balance, alternating the strokes until simultaneously mastering the slash stroke and balance control.

Decrease or increase the height of the sack, in order to practice the blows at different heights, releasing the impact from different angles, always very quickly, immediately returning the foot to its place.

I repeat, the blow must be very fast, dry and strong, followed by a push, taking care to keep the balance, returning the foot quickly to its place of departure; all this in a fraction of seconds.

I place special emphasis on keeping your balance at all costs, since a good shot is useless if you lose, even momentarily, the plumb balance that we need to maintain during skirmishes; try the above hundreds of times, make sure your eyes do not indicate your intentions otherwise; The practice will teach you to know before the execution, the movement that the opposite plans, this can be guessed in the look, in the way of standing in front of you, therefore, I recommend studying these small, at the same time great details , which are the basis of success in Karate.

Mastering the blow with the foot is of capital importance, as will be seen later, when we enter into sets that require the use of this resource; therefore, it is necessary to learn it thoroughly.

Karate punch with the tips of the fingers of the hand

A great resource of this sport is to use the tips of the fingers of the hands to deliver a sharp and localized blow on a vulnerable point.

Study carefully the graph, in which a hand appears training on a Makiwara and against a sack; This training can be done indistinctly against one or the other, the interesting thing is to do it well.

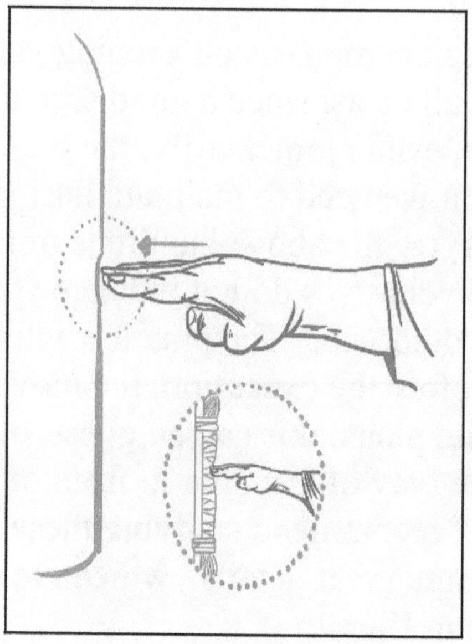

The classics advise doing the initial workouts by sticking with the tips of the fingers in a container with lentils, sawdust, etc.

Which will move to the sides allowing your hand to slide between them.

I recommend this practice against the sack, first with little force, barely touching it, increasing the blow in force as your fingers harden and withstand the impacts; When your hand has hardened in the blows you will notice that your fingers are stronger and more resistant and your blows more and more accurate.

At that moment we will begin to look for aim,
directing the blows with surveyor's accuracy, to
the points where they should hit; such points are
illustrated in the following graph.

As you can see, it is about the eyes, the nut of
the throat, the neck in general, as well as the soft
parts of the abdomen.

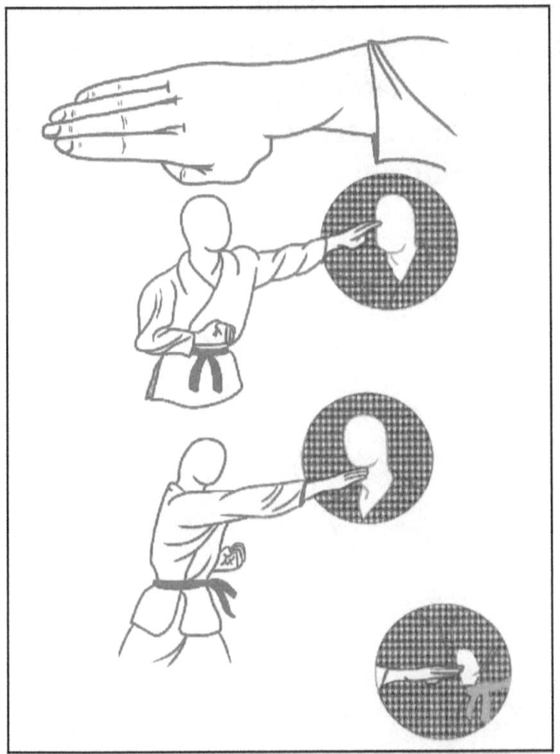

This blow is brutal when done well; its results,
depending on where it hits the target, are
overwhelming.

Therefore, I recommend caution for your
training, and your practice against a partner
should be closely watched to avoid injury.

In short, the practice of this blow should be done exactly the same as the one I indicated for learning the corkscrew blow with a closed fist, because in this case there is no possibility of injuring the hand, although the blow does promote possible injuries to the fingers. which can range from a simple twist to a fracture; Therefore, I insist on taking things calmly, previously hardening the hand with hand preparation exercises and then gradually taking the training against something hard.

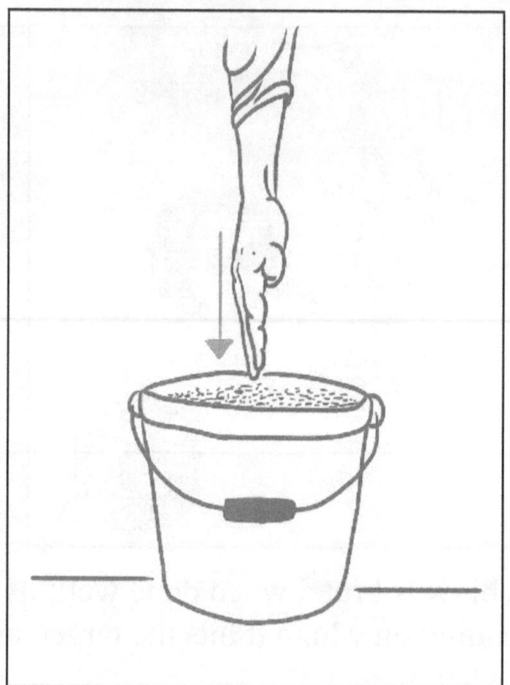

Achieving this blow takes a long time, at least a year, hence the reader will have to gather a lot of patience and work slowly, but without rest, hardening his hands, fingers and wrists, to be able to count in his repertoire of blows this effective knowledge.

When the blow described is directed to the eyes of the opponent, the fingers should open in a V, two for each side, little finger and ring finger together to one side, and the middle finger with the index to the opposite side, forming a letter V.

We must take care of this blow, since its results alone prove its dangerousness.

The following figure shows us a strange training method, which consists of using a container full of lentils, where the hand is stuck like a knife; This serves to harden the fingers, preparing them to be used in this unique Karate resource.

Karate Heel Strike

I present to my readers another Karate resource, which consists of using the heel; for this it is also necessary to harden said part of the foot, preparing it to deliver heavy blows.

In the graph I present the way to train this blow, which can be done against the Makiwara of which we have been talking so much, or use the boxer's training bag; Both will help the reader to achieve punch, give strength and hardness to his heel so that it stoically withstands impacts and can be used later as a weapon.

This blow is given with force, carrying with it all the weight of the body; it is executed quickly, seeking aim without losing balance, or off balance, immediately picking up the leg to bring it to its starting point, all of which must be done in a fraction of a second.

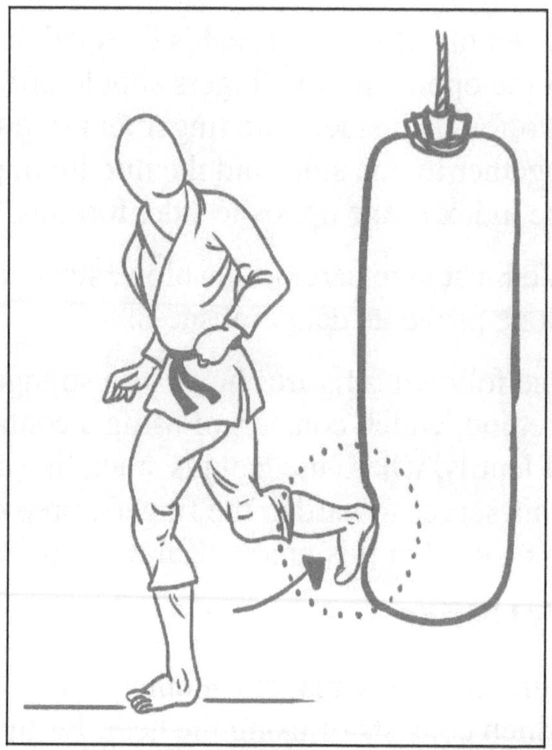

The trajectory of the blow must be diagonal, studied, elegant, without confusing it with a vulgar parry, but rather as a perfectly calculated thrust that will carry, as previously noted, great force in its impact and accurate aim; Therefore, we will begin from this moment its practice until we achieve a perfect mastery of this stroke.

Dear reader, be your own and most demanding judge, diligently watching your movements, first in front of a mirror, then in shadow, and finally, roughly hitting the sack; If you consider that you have already learned one hundred percent, this blow, then we can go through the chapter, not before, as it would be harmful.

Remember that executing a karate blow badly done or badly learned is as much as not knowing it.

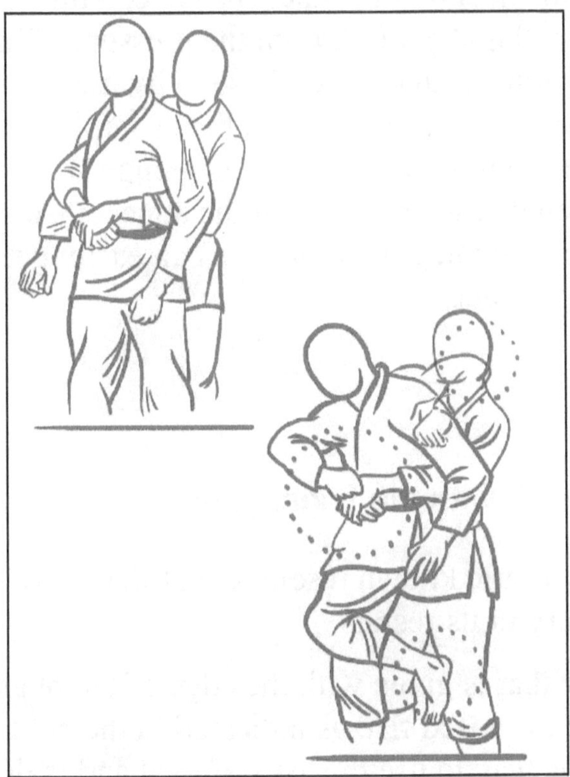

Now we will go on to use the previous knowledge in a practical way, using it as a means to get out of the grip, with which the graph is illustrated, in which, as the reader can appreciate, it serves as an open sesame to release the grip.

Let us study the drawings in the aforementioned graph carefully and move to the training mat to practice the counter grip and its exit, taking advantage of two Karate blows delivered with the heel on the attacker's knee, with which we will make him loosen the pressure of his arms , moment that we will use to by means of a waist twist, first to the front, then sharply to the side, to loosen or semi-loosen enough so that with the elbow, we roughly hit the attacker's lower maximal, with which we can easily get out of his embrace .

Karate punch with the finger joints

Karate has a little known resource, but like all of this sport, extraordinary in its results.

It is a blow that is given with the edge of the phalanges, with the semi-closed fist, as indicated in the next graphic, in which the way to use this part of the hand is drawn to deliver sharp blows concentrated in neuralgically points weak.

Well, this blow, because of how rare it is in itself, requires even more adequate study if you want to obtain the returns for which they were designed.

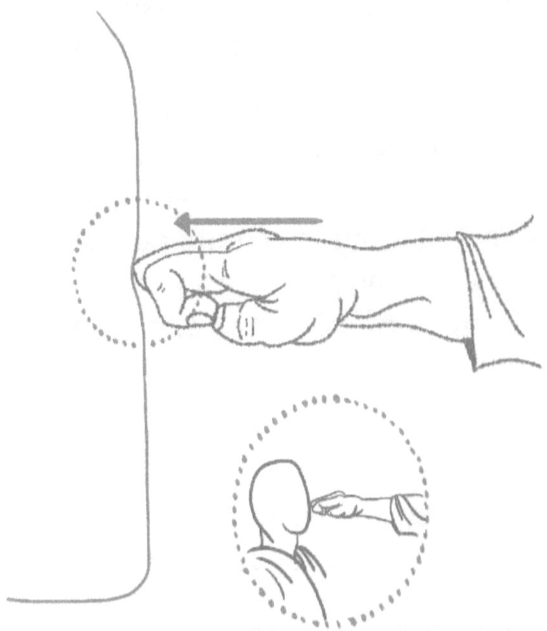

His training requires the same recommended guidelines for the above strokes, that is, his practice must be done against the Makiwara or against the training bag, which is precisely what I recommend.

To begin, one must learn to present the hand by putting it heavily armed, with the fingers bent, presenting the knuckles of the phalanges in front; the thumb will be bent over the fingernails, ensuring its proper posture; the blow is given in a straight way, following a form similar to what in boxing is called jab or right cross; its main objective is to crash against the base of the nose, or against the teeth; its impacts are withering, as they destroy.

Your training must always be increasing, forcing you to withstand greater and greater impacts, as you notice that your hand is hardening and holding this training train.

This is not a forcefully devastating blow like the one with the clenched fist, it is used to harass weak points.

As you have to learn it well, I recommend practicing first as usual, in front of a mirror, then with shadow exercises, looking for ease, placement and style, and finally, I recommend training by hitting to acquire punch in this regard; I must clarify that the punch is a gift of nature with which some people are born, but it can be achieved through constant blows against the sack.

Now I recommend that my readers go to their training place and put into practice the training of this stroke, until they have it well executed and perfectly assimilated to their wealth of new knowledge about our sport.

Give me a lever and a fulcrum and I'll move the world

Get up, have breakfast, study or go to work, come back and do holds, squats, biceps work to the gym; Surely he repeats this every day, that is, to train, right? But what would you think if I told you that the reason why gyms were designed is something completely different from what it is today.

To better express this concept, we are going to break down the word gym.

From the Greek word gymnasium means a place to go naked.

The word could be said to be a temple where people liberate or find their soul in order to grow.

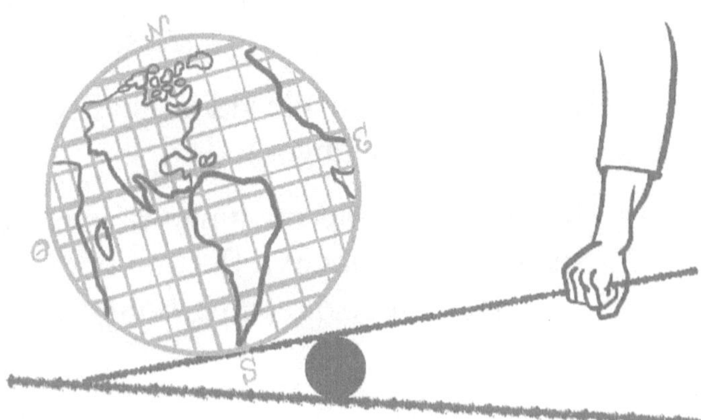

The word gymnasium of ancient Greece and describe a place of sports, arts and science in ancient times, no matter how humble, that can contribute to cultivate their physique shares of education of young people also in these complexes that include subjects to exercise both the body, as well as the teaching of music, grammar, philosophy and painting.

Many gymnasiums had a library, in fact it is usually surrounded by large gardens where the disciples listened to the philosophers' teachers.

But the gym was much more than a place to do sports, it was also a meeting place to be able to talk about what is spiritually and above all to become wiser to obtain a lot of knowledge, perhaps by this term from ancient Greece; children and boys followed a philosophy and took great care of their bodies.

Procuring a valuable aid to intellectual formation as they are no longer today.

It was a very important part of everyday life, since people sought reflection not only doing exercises but also reading, studying, composing, observing.

Obviously these are other times and this has changed a lot ...

Most athletes in the gym only depend on it as a physical space and the machines that make it up, it is also just limited to following instructions taking a little learning and tools to build their physique as people.

A division has been created where the muscular ones criticize the intellectuals and the intellectuals the muscular ones; when history shows that the one who lifts weights was as capable as the one who flips through books.

For example, muscle is very good, but if for example you realize that I check it, they can help you avoid injuries when lifting a heavy load, in your daily life or protect the wrong forces when exercising, strength to perform better, just imagine Now in these moments that an intellectual will not happen to you, or for example a book that tells you what to do properly.

How to take advantage of your body?

You know how to take advantage of that place only with their current knowledge if you look through history these people who went to the gyms did not go only for the physical space, but for the knowledge and guidance of the teachers.

Evolution; I am like we no longer write on papyri, current cases are not learning centers like today it is difficult to imagine gyms that house space for poets, doctors, musicians, if the history of the gym began like this, how would you imagine the future of gyms ...

Due to quarantines or people's beliefs, today the gyms have been closed indefinitely, we do not know if they will be the same ...

Perhaps thanks to input holograms that do not have the shape as the machines that we already know need, they will continue to evolve and applications will triple in number.

In what way do you imagine the future then?

Inside the house, everyone wants to set up a gym, and they think they should buy machines, mats, etc. ...

When really a gym is both a sports place, as that place you take to talk, read, write, etc. If you wonder what a real gym is like, it is enough to understand that those who only compose music, or draw, and those who lift several kilos exercise both, therefore, it is not impossible to put a Dojo, Temple, or less a Gym at home .

Our part, dear reader, will be that we will keep the concept of the real gym alive and it is not simply a utopia to work in a culture that not only enters the muscles, but also to think about the way it moves, be it with its body the knowledge of personal tastes as an exercise of the mind and it is in time of its complicity process exposed by us and if your important passion is for the most important machine; our body the true temple.

Whoever says, "I don't have time to go to the gym" should have time to look around ...

Flying Kick (Authentic)

I present to the readers this exciting resource of our sport that is illustrated in the drawing of the next graphic.

Its realization requires great agility, constant training and feline speed.

In purely sporting matches, it is used to give the skirmish color and joy, especially some completely "unreal" ones.

It is not advisable to use it as personal defense or in street fights, since its results could be counterproductive.

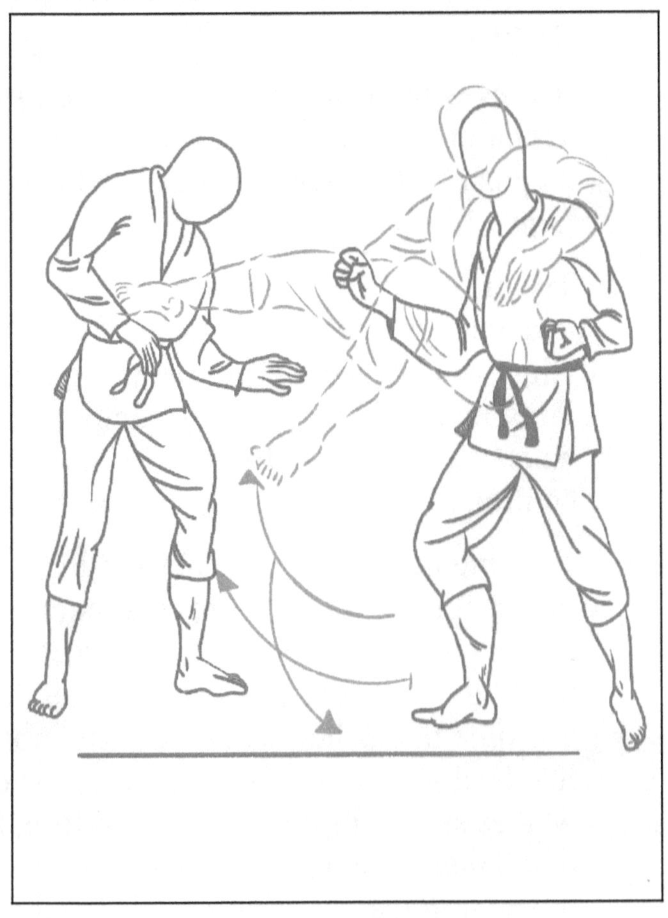

To master the true flying kick, you must train in front of the sack, following the following guidelines: Slightly advance the leg to be struck; jump, as high as possible, throw the kick with a sudden movement, which will emanate precisely from the hips; Lean your body back slightly, hit the marked target, and immediately fall on your guard.

It goes without saying that it can be called a kangaroo kick because it is mainly taking a jump by pushing the waist, foot or feet towards the target, like a lunge.

Trying to fall standing in the precise place he had when leaving; I cushioned the fall with a slight bend of the knee to the front, springing the fall with the thighs, thereby controlling his balance, making the balance remain in absolute control.

Jumping heights helps to master this resource that is not easy to achieve, as it requires, like all karate movements, long years of tedious training, but it is worth it because all the sweat and time that is burned in the gym , translates into health, physical and mental well-being as well as sports improvement; therefore, I recommend that my readers start from this moment in learning this knowledge that will pay such useful dividends.

Let's start practicing in front of the mirror, then we'll go on to shadow training, practicing alone, in order to achieve the necessary style and speed; from there to hitting training against the sack, looking for aim and precision, and only when this resource is well assimilated, will we begin to practice it against a partner in learning skirmishes.

As a last recommendation, there is to keep your mouth tightly closed. So, let's move immediately to our gym and start the referred practice.

THE TOTAL AND CORRECT ASSIMILATION OF THE LANCES OF THE CHAPTERS THAT COME NEXT, REQUIRE A LOT OF PATIENCE.

Remember that:

"Patience is the mother of all sciences."

Karate Strike Training

Illustrated in the graph are four karate punches that are trained against a boxing practice bag.

Karate classics do this training against a Makiwara, but I find more advantages in the sack, so I recommend it, although I depart from the traditional canons.

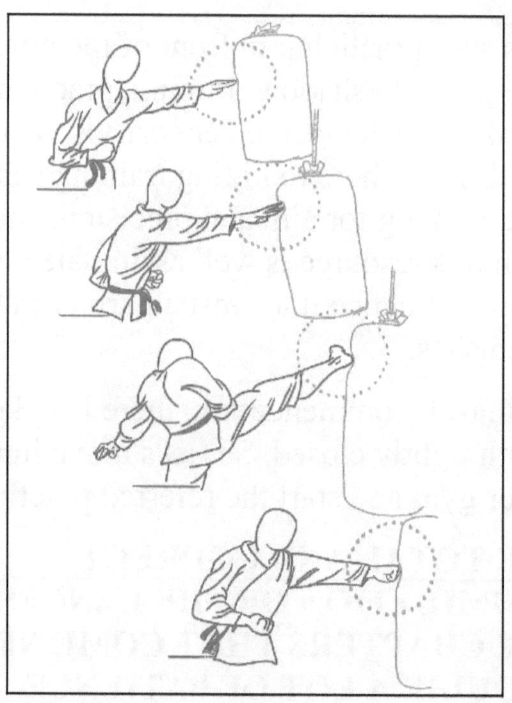

The main advantages are: that the sack has volume, weight, mobility, human shape, as well as that it is an accessory that can easily be purchased in sporting goods stores.

Well, whether against one or another accessory, the important thing is to train with strength and perseverance the knowledge that in this small treatise I detail.

The first days of practice you should hit lightly, looking for ease, aim, and settlement; As their fingers, hands and feet get used to it and stiffen, the hitting will get harder, setting their impacts more solidly, taking care not to injure themselves.

Some aspirants, in their initial voracity logic, rush, thereby obtaining fractures, dislocations, etc .; For this reason I recommend the reader to go slowly, but without pause, hardening little by little.

Let's remember that a karate expert requires a minimum of five years of constant training to mature.

After the previous recommendations, we move in front of the sack and we will begin our practices.

The upper figure shows the blow that is delivered with the tips of the fingers, which is directed against the most vulnerable points of the opponent, such as the eyes and the solar plexus, so that the training in the sack will be against drawings of these places that we have made in it so that our training is directed precisely to those points.

The second figure from top to bottom, bears the opponent's eyes as an indication and white; the blow is given with the middle and ring fingers open in a "V" shape.

This blow is definitive because of its tremendous roughness, you have to practice it a lot to obtain ease in the placement of the fingers, which, with a simple movement, should remain open, forming exactly the letter "V", aided by the little finger that will stick to the ring, on the one hand, and on the other the index that will strengthen the central or middle finger; The blow will carry the characteristic of a lunge, with the movement that occurs in boxing to the blow known as the right cross, with that arm, or jab with the left arm.

I recommend taking great care of your style, so that this shot comes out flawless, being prudent in your training and constantly practicing in front of the mirror.

Now we will go on to train the kick illustrated in the following drawing from top to bottom. It appears drawn in the classic sporting way of using this resource, which targets the solar plexus of the opponent, of course there are more vulnerable places, such as the testicles; train in front of the mirror first to learn how to stand on one leg; achieved this first fundamental aspect, go to train against the sack; the blow must carry motive force, emanating from the hips.

It is not an ordinary kick that is done by throwing the foot, our karate movement starts, as previously noted, from the hip, because that is what gives strength to its impacts; the blow must be like lightning in its speed; as soon as it hits the target, it will return to its place of departure.

This throw must be surprising, accurate in its aim and extraordinarily fast, having to carry 60% of our body weight when crashing to give greater force to the impact.

Finally, we will study the blow that appears outlining in the figure below, which is delivered with a closed fist, setting the knuckles against the sack; this blow must hit the opponent's face or chest, targets that must be painted on the sack to achieve aim during training.

This devastating blow leaves the guard position, placing the fist more or less at the waist, from there it shoots forward by twisting the arm, describing a corkscrew movement inwards, so that when it reaches its destination, the palm of the hand points down; the shoulder muscles should be relaxed; wrist and forearm.

I repeat, the fist, in its place of departure, will point the palm of the hand upwards, during the trajectory it will make the corkscrew movement, so that when reaching the target the palm of the hand points downwards; With the impulse of the blow, rotate your hips, loading 60% of your weight on your arm; To increase the power of the punch, strike with the knuckles of the index and middle fingers and return immediately to your original starting position.

With the previous explanations begin your daily practice, seeking each time to hit with greater aim, precision and force.

Consistency in training will give you the indispensable punch, being recommended to bandage hands and wrists for the first months, to avoid dislocations; It is also convenient to practice this blow in front of the mirror, in order to correct your position, not forgetting to do constant shadow training in order to obtain style, ease, a sense of balance, distance and speed.

Locks

A very important phase is learning to block blows, deflecting them with forearm blows.

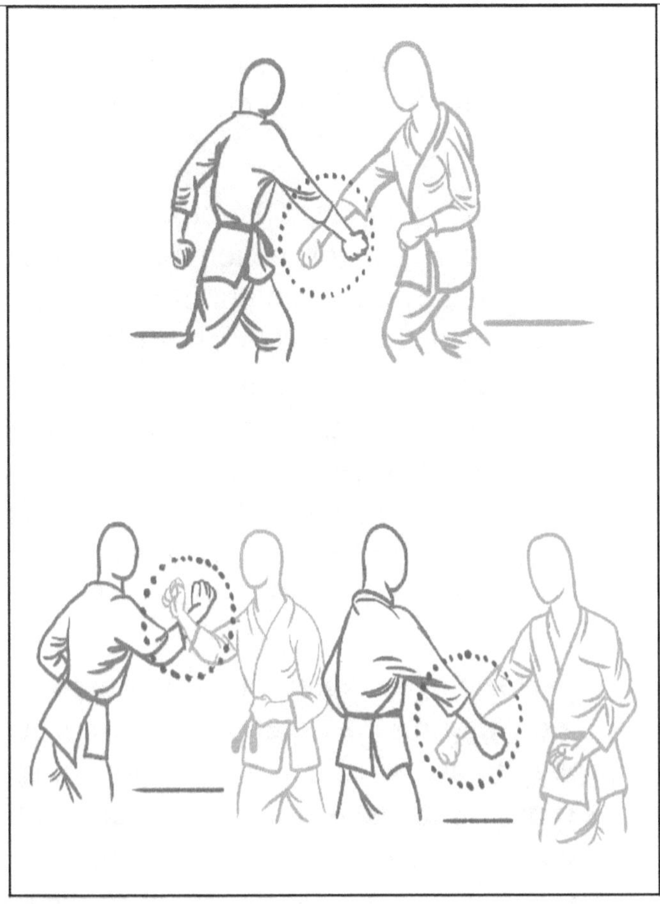

These resources are illustrated in the drawings of the graph, which we will study in detail in theory, in which its purpose is easily appreciated, which is to deflect direct blows to the body, which are blocked before they reach their destination.

This training is quite rough, it hurts the forearms the first few times, but its constant practice manages to harden the muscles, making the painful sensation somewhat lose; it certainly does not make the student Fakir.

But it makes you lose the fear of pain by creating a healthy routine that hardens muscles and mind to such a degree that pain goes almost unnoticed.

Well, let's first train the blocking movements in front of the mirror, which will always be followed by a movement of deflection towards the outside of the opponent's blow; When these blocks work out well in the mirror, we will go on to train them in the shade, seeking to perform the movements very quickly; From there we will go on to practice against the sack, in order to accustom our forearms to impacts, and finally, the training will be formal, against a partner, the first times carrying the block or blocks to be performed by default, marking in movements In slow motion the exact place of impact and the way to use force laterally, to deflect the blow by tying, so to speak, on the contrary with the continuous blocking-push, which immediately opens a large gap in the guard of the attacker.

When the exact blocking place has been found, we will begin the practice increasing the force, the speed and the impacts.

Finally, we will carry out the training with the roughness necessary to fully familiarize ourselves with the roughness of this beautiful sport.

It is convenient that in this type of training partners of different sizes, weights, reflexes, etc., alternate so that the blank is more complete, since it is not advantageous to always use the same partner, since we would take the measurement in a few workouts , thereby falling into a routine of equal reflexes; In addition, it is advisable to train on the most varied sites: flat, inclined, rough, slippery, wet, etc., to accustom our reflexes to react strongly on any terrain and against any opponent.

With the above recommendations, continue your workouts.

Karate placement and technical movements

One of the fundamental elements of any sport is to be able to walk moving intelligently; in ours, moving properly is basic, therefore, this chapter will be dedicated to studying the ideal form of positioning and movements aimed at achieving a refined sporting style that facilitates the substantial development of throws, blows, blocks, etc., which you need to know and master a karate player to perfection.

In the graph, the figure of one of the primary aspects is illustrated, which is to be well standing, firmly supported on the soles of the feet, working in a balanced position, with the spring of the muscles ready to work.

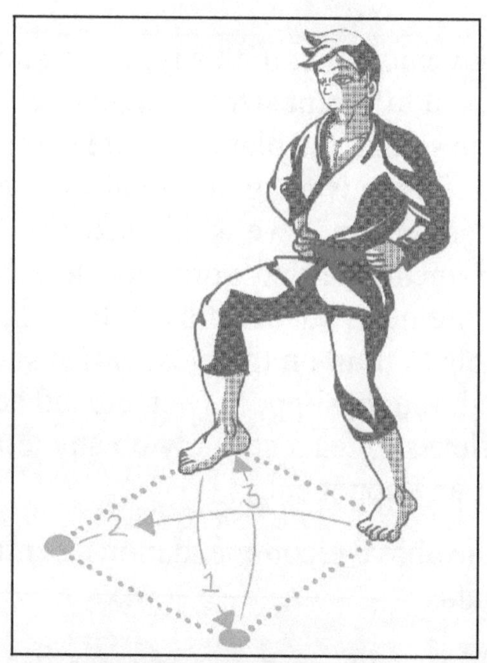

Upon achieving the above, we will begin their learning in front of a mirror, moving slowly, changing the position of the feet as indicated by the numbers and arrows; The distance that should be between one leg and another will fluctuate according to their height, but it will be approximately sixty centimeters, and they should never join, as this would cause them to lose balance and stumble; the muscles will be slightly contracted to have spring; the movements will be harmonious, coordinated, slow during the first days, seeking to find exactly the right position.

Once this has been achieved, we will try to make the movements increasingly rapid, that they do not involve efforts that become normal within their way of walking, this last point being very important, since their movements must be made with the ease of a reflex, without think to run it.

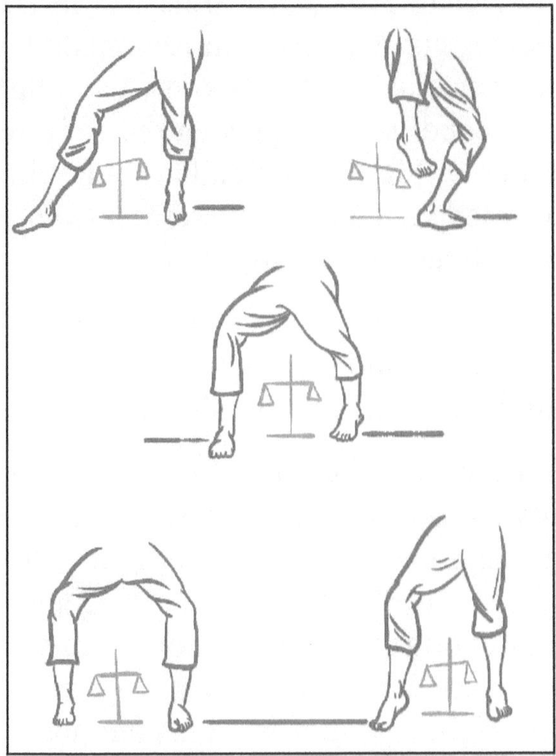

When the above has been achieved, we will go on to study the figures that illustrate the graph, in which some of the tactical movements of Karate appear, tending to approach the target, retreat, seek support for a blow, etc.

In all these movements the vital thing is to move transferring the weight of your body from one leg to the other, without altering the balance that your balance must keep; The practice of these movements should be done not only on a level and hard ground, but it should be practiced on any type of ground, regardless of its shape, uneven, cut, inclined, uneven, muddy, dusty, etc., since in We do not know the future under what conditions or on what type of terrain the reader will have to defend himself with his knowledge of Karate; therefore, we must learn to move intelligently anywhere.

After working in front of the mirror, when his movements look normal and his reflexes are quick, we will rehearse shadow workouts.

Starting from the starting position, start your forward position practice, which is done by bringing your left leg forward for a distance of approximately one meter, bearing about half your own weight; the toes of the forward foot will point a bit inwards, which gives stability, your right leg will carry the contracted muscles, it will be ready to move also to the front if necessary; keep your balance perfectly distributed, the movement of the leg in front should emanate from your hips, firmly, quickly and decisively; do not drag your leg, throw it with great speed, because in this lies the difference in movements that our sport has.

Your body will remain; slightly back so as not to present white.

When you have learned the forward movements well, let's practice the backward movement, which is exactly the same in terms of study, with the difference that this is also done with hip movements, but backwards.

Let's practice this movement as many times as necessary in front of the mirror, so that it serves as a judge and criticizes these movements if they come out correct or not.

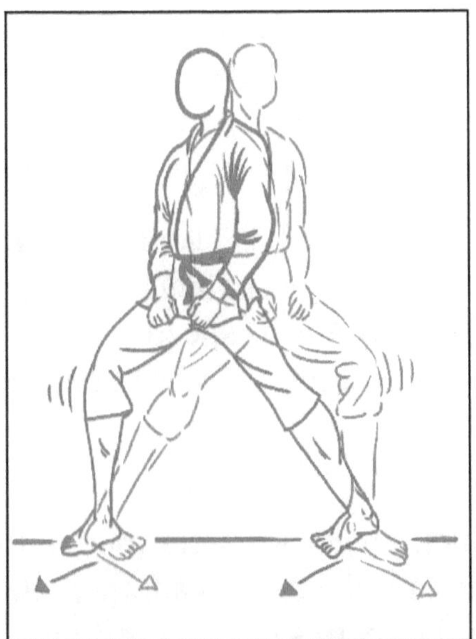

Let us remember once again that the movements of the legs are made with rapid movements that emanate from the hips, that the toes should point inwards for greater support.

Finally, we will study the change of direction or pivot.

This in itself is a movement of the right flank or of the left flank, which consists of advancing or delaying a leg, making a quick turn on that foot that allows us to immediately change lateral position, rounding this practice with twisting movements of the waist, tending to facilitate such movements.

Practice turning by sliding your feet on the ground as in military march training, which forces you to change the direction of the flanks, either with half-turn or flanking exercises; With the above we will have learned the movements towards the front, backwards, pivot or change of direction to the right and to the left, as well as the twisting of the waist of the upper part of the body from the hips up.

With this I conclude this chapter, but not without first recommending its exhaustive practice until achieving extraordinary speed, great coordination, absolute sense of balance, muscular control and spring.

After assimilating one hundred percent of the above, which gives us a solid foundation, we are in a position to move on to another chapter to delve into the secrets of this exciting sport.

The guard

The position or positions that place the performer in a suitable situation are identified with the name of guard, which facilitates the free movement of their body towards defensive positions, at the same time that they make the path to an attack clear; This attack is of great importance in sports such as boxing, judo, wrestling, etc., and in our Karate it could not be less, so we are going to carefully study the most usual guard positions, in order to adopt those that more accommodate the reader, taking into account their idiosyncrasies and the special characteristics of their physique.

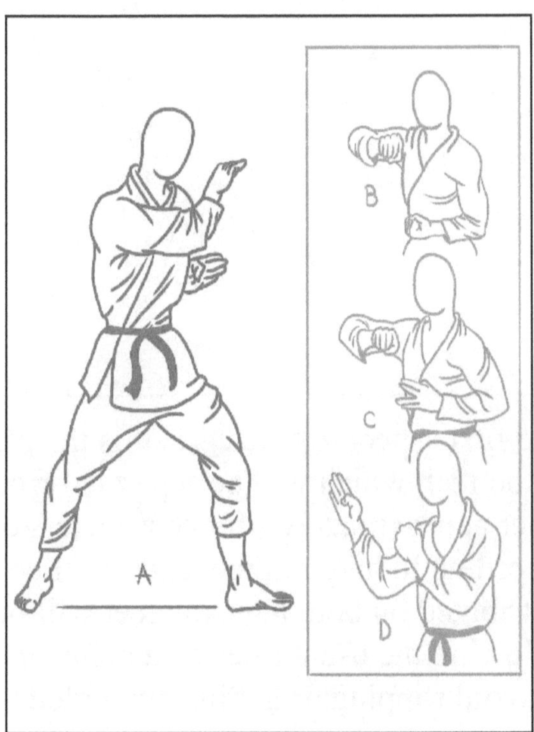

Entering the subject, we will begin by carefully observing the illustrations in the following graphs, where nine possible guard positions are drawn; these are adapted to almost all the needs of sports guards and for contingencies of street encounters.

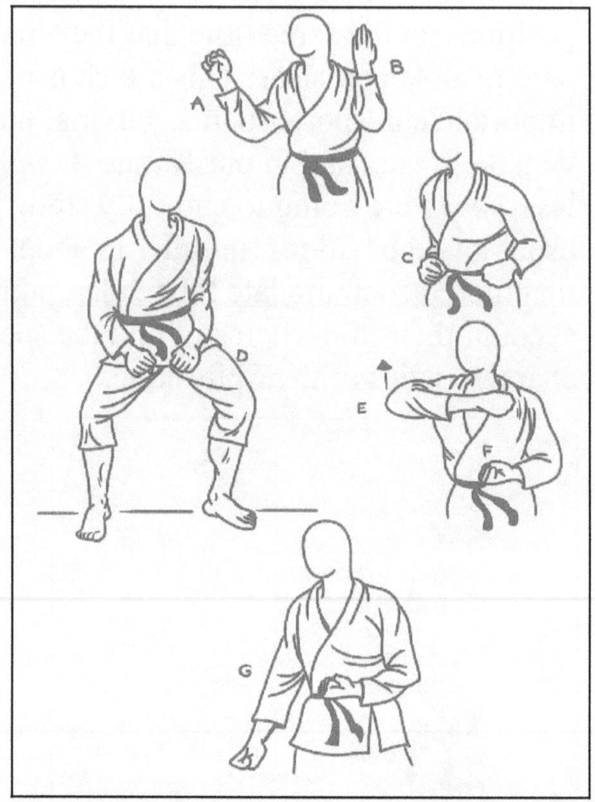

The first aspect to take care of is the placement of the feet, which will be separated from each other approximately fifty centimeters or more, according to height; the weight will be evenly distributed on both legs, the feet will be moved following the usual rules of fencing and boxing, to avoid tripping or getting entangled with them.

The movement to the front, back and to the sides must be fluid (this I have dealt with in full in its corresponding chapter), the arms will be placed in a defensive position carrying the hand armed with the blow that is planned to give, of course without telegraphing to the contrary your intention with the placement of your hands.

In sports matches, on the contrary, by simply seeing the shape their hands take, they can already imagine and foresee the possible attack, but in street encounters with laymen in the field, the reader will have a considerable advantage, since the ignorance of our techniques of Combat will make the form of attack that we will shoot unpredictable and, logically, it will not have elements of adequate defense against our weapons.

The figure marked with the letter "A" shows a guard posture armed with a slash; This position is ideal for preventing an armed attack. The position marked with the letter "B" is designed to block a blow diagonally against the head with a blunt object.

The letter "C" guard is roughly the same as the previous one, but his left hand is armed with V-shaped fingers ready to counterattack.

The guard that appears illustrated in the figure of the letter "D", is a common position, which allows the immediate attack with the open hand, with the tips of the fingers; These guards are quite practical, they are generally used in sports-type skirmishes.

Now we will go on to study the guard of the same graph, starting with the drawing of the letter "E", which shows how to get into a normal position, although in a defensive attitude, with the muscles of the thighs contracted, with the spring ready to go, arms ready for immediate action; This attitude does not impose, however, it is basic in this sport.

Let's enter the study of the figure marked with the letter "F", which is adopting a defensive attitude with his hands armed with the chop. The figure illustrated with the letter "G", is more or less the same as the previous one, varying only in the presentation of the hands, which on occasion are presented with the fist firmly closed and, consequently, the attack will be with another type of hit.

Let us now analyze the guard of the figure marked with the letter "H"; in this position it is the elbow that appears threatening, with the opposite fist ready to strike with the knuckles; and finally, we have the figure of the position illustrated with the letter "J", in which the clenched fists appear, one cocked and the other in a speculative position, but ready to be fired; These guards are used the same in the right natural guard as in the opposite or left-handed guard, taking into account the natural disposition of the reader.

These guards are, as I previously noted, fundamentally defensive considering the possible attack that they need to stop, their second aspect being that of setting a trap for the opposite by engulfing it by apparently offering an easy target of a vital point of our body, which we will learn from beforehand so that when it is thrown against us, we make it fall into a counter blow, as one would say in boxing, that is, hit it while receiving it, with which the power of our blow will be increased.

Once the previous guard positions have been outlined, we will move in front of a mirror to begin our learning and we will take those that fully satisfy us, discarding those that do not fit their type.

After executing them well in front of the mirror, we will practice them intensely in the shade, seeking to turn them into natural reflections.

Finally, we will take them to formal practice in skirmishes with a partner in front of us, seeking to polish them by making them more perfect each occasion in their operation and performance, combining them as much as necessary.

Practice is the one that will most intelligently advise the reader which or which are the ideal guards.

Of course, the first skirmishes will only be "marking" the blow without making impacts. And in these marking trainings, we will refine what we previously learned in theory.

Look to switch training partners to maximize your focus.

Combat tactics

Now I will teach the reader an extraordinary secret of a psychological nature, which also provides great physical ease; I am referring to a loud and guttural scream that occurs unexpectedly when attacking and that brings as logical consequences a confusion in the opponent; If he is profane in the matter, his bewilderment will be even greater, since normally, anyone who hears a loud scream will go out of his mind if this turn is uttered precisely at a time when his nerves are in tension: The result it will be a total mismatch in fractions of a second, which should be used intelligently to attack through the gap that it leaves open.

It is necessary to have this cry well rehearsed for it to produce the desired effect, therefore, it should also be a reason for special training.

In addition, when emitting this cry, the immediate attack will be synchronized, in order to make the most of the confusion that, as I said before, is created in the opponent's mind; The reader should not underestimate this great combat tactic, since its performances are fabulous, because in addition to the confusion described, the scream brings with it a very important physical aspect, which increases the force of our blows, since when screaming, striking simultaneously We are letting the air escape from our lungs, which, when contained in the pre-attack, gives us greater vigor when striking.

This is easy to verify: If we observe the movements of specialist weightlifting athletes, we will see that when they fill their lungs they pull the weights upwards, being that deep oxygen inspiration the one that provides them with the necessary help for the effort To make; after this, the air is released.

Now, the most commonly used cry is similar to the one used by muleteers to stop their horses and that is a sound that resembles "Yan", so that, from today, my readers should use this novel resource when training; When the blows are practiced, when making impact, emit your battle cry to gradually adapt to its use and achieve more and more stridency.

Let's synchronize the scream and breathing in our chopping workouts, to give greater force to the blow; This is not easy to achieve, since a lot of training is required, combining the aforementioned aspects, which are: The contained breath, the blow and the scream all in unison; Compare your impacts before and after you gain this knowledge and keep training intensely until you achieve perfection.

You can change the scream for a loud whistle, which stuns the opponent's eardrum, and draws attention in case of street; although it is more difficult to practice.

To neutralize the opponent's arms

In the graph, a very simple resource is drawn to neutralize the opponent's arms; Let's study the aforementioned drawing in detail and move to our training mat to practice it exhaustively.

It is finished off with a violent karate blow with the elbow, over the opponent's ear. This cast is used against an opponent dressed, but with the jacket or jacket unbuttoned it consists, as the drawing indicates, in imprisoning his arms by surprise, tying them, as it were, with the same jacket, which we will semi remove at a height of approximately ten inches more below their shoulders, solidly holding the clothing to prevent it from being repositioned, thereby losing effect on the cast.

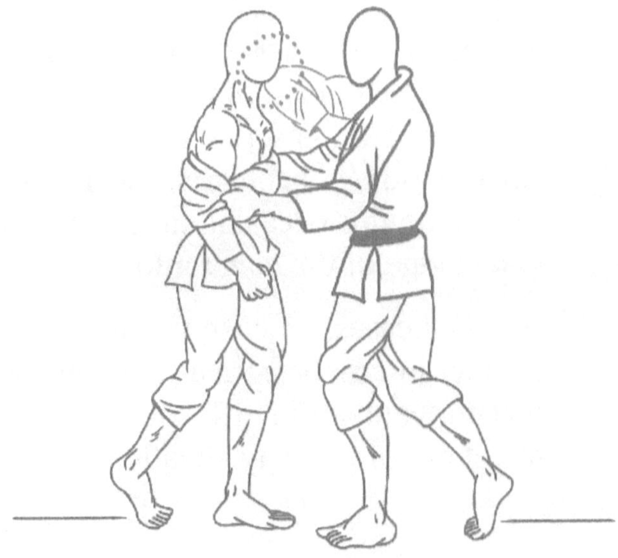

To avoid this, synchronize the movements of lowering the bag, with a ruthless elbow against your ear, or precisely in the place of union, where the upper and lower maximillae make vertex, since this is an extremely vulnerable place; hence the opponent is completely stunned by the blow or blows, in addition to imprisoning with his own clothing.

Entering the subject, you must first become familiar with the drawing, understand it well in theory and with your skirmish partner take it to practice as many times as necessary, until it is fully assimilated.

During training, teammates should alternate, sometimes as attacked, sometimes as attackers, practicing the counter and the corresponding block (s), in order to perfectly learn one thing and another and be able to execute them with all cleanliness and opportunity.

The counter to this set is the same one that is used to free ourselves from an attack against the throat, which I describe in full in the corresponding chapter, and which it is advisable to read on this occasion to round off the knowledge of the counter to this set.

As in all cases, I advise you to practice this counter intensely from all possible angles, placing yourself in different postures, to be able to get out of it in any situation.

To let go of a grip on our wrists

Let's study the following graph, which illustrates how to easily let go of any grip on our wrists.

At the top there is a two-handed shot of our wrist; to get away, turn the wooden fist so that your fingers point upwards, lower your elbow a few centimeters, make force with your wrist attacking the opponent's thumbs, which are the weak part of your hand, pull against them and your wrist will be free.

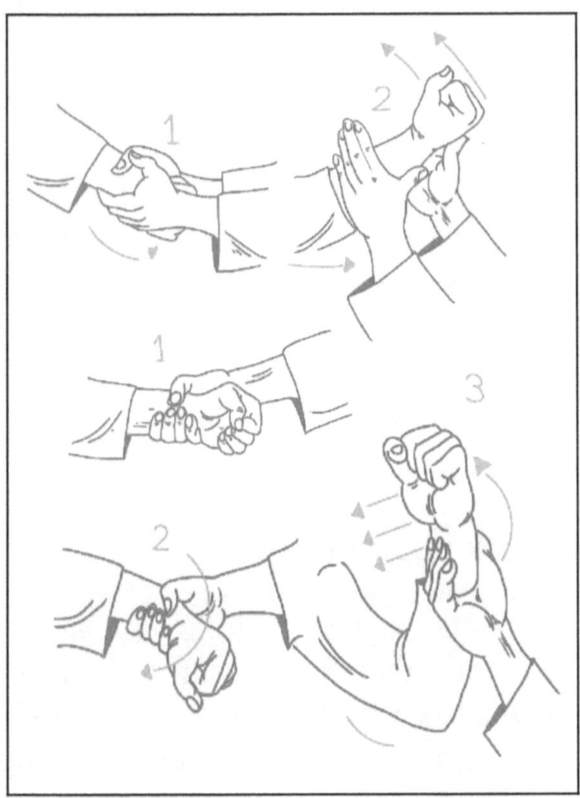

At the bottom there are three drawings that deal with a one-handed grip on our wrists; Study the second movement, which consists of turning the fist with force, in order to place ourselves in a position that allows the normal movement of the arm illustrated by figure number 3, which refers to how to get rid of the grip, making an attack

I want to establish the above, as an antecedent of the way in which the force intelligently directed against the point or points that at a given moment are the weak ones should be used; in the present case, the opponent's hand is the source on the side where the four fingers are located and offers a hole on the side of the thumb.

Practice the previous recommendations, observing what is indicated in the relative graphs and of course place yourself in all kinds of imaginable positions, in order that you learn to get out of those grips, no matter the situation in which you are placed.

Practice will give you the exact pattern to follow to become proficient in this outing.

Defensive block and slash attack

In the drawings in the following graph, I present a skirmish that illustrates how to block a boxing blow known as the right crusader, giving the appropriate response by roughly hitting the opponent's kidneys and lower ribs, with a slash blow of the left hand.

Look carefully at the above drawings and we will immediately move on to your formal practice. My recommendations are as follows: When blocking, I forcefully deflected the right hand outward, hitting the opponent's hard with his forearm, follow the impact of the blow with a push, as I indicated above, outward, as this will momentarily take the player off balance. attacker, moments that we will use to hit his kidneys and lower ribs as roughly as possible; When you do this, stay alert to continue attacking more vulnerable points, such as the neck and neck, or return your body to a defensive guard position.

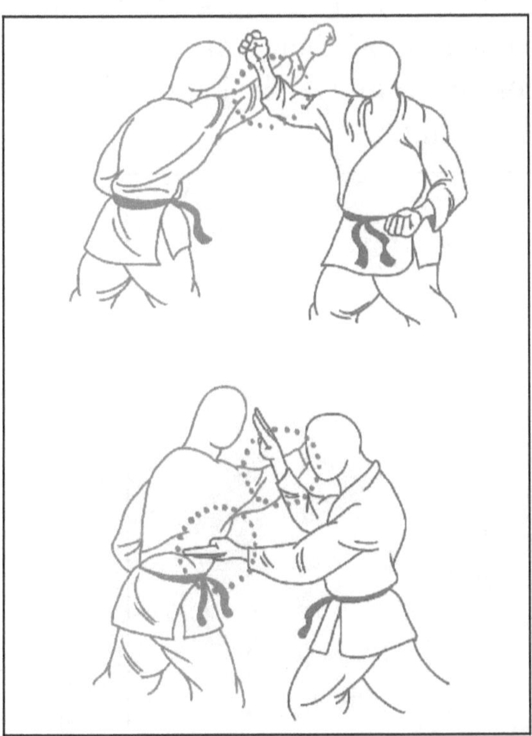

Practice this block as many times as you think necessary, until it is sufficiently assimilated to be easily performed in true attacks. Of course, you should not underestimate the ability of the opponent in them, nor do you feel overly confident; always be ready, with your intelligence wide awake to defend yourself with all the necessary malice.

When you master this set to perfection, we will move on from chapter

Defensive block and kick attack

Now we will study the graph, in which it is illustrated how to block a boxing blow known by the name of jab, being the counterattack that I recommend to use, the karate blow that is tipped with the foot.

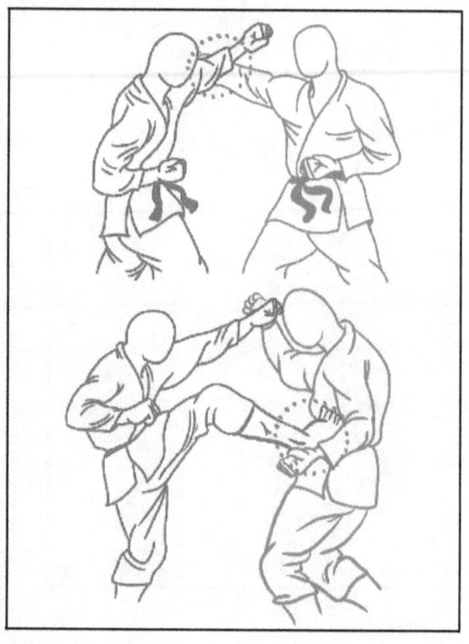

Let's take a close look at the classic form of this cast and get ready to take it to your training, following the directions below:

Wait for the blow in a defensive guard position; As the latter comes forward with your left arm with a closed fist, counter by striking the opponent's forearm with your own.

Continue this blow with a push of the aforementioned forearm outwards, to deflect the blow, and at the same time, open the guard of your opponent, taking him off balance; When doing this, kick hard to the stomach, if it's a friendly sparring, or to the testicles if it's self-defense, in a true attack.

The way of kicking is already well known to the reader, but I will review it anyway. Raise your knee as high as possible, from there throw the kick to the front, leaving said movement of the hips carrying 60% of the weight of your body after the kick, so that its impact is forceful; immediately return the leg to its place of departure; if the blow was accurate and hit the target, subsequent success will be in your hands.

At this point the reader will have enough training, speed and malice to determine the type of attack to follow, as well as the karate blows to use.

As in all sets, this one needs to be practiced hundreds of times, with all kinds of partners, tall, thick, short, etc., in order to achieve the necessary blank.

Do your practices on uneven terrain, to be sufficiently trained and be able to defend yourself on any terrain.

Defensive Block and Fist Attack

Now we will study how to counterattack using the most forceful and devastating blow in karate. In the graph where it appears illustrated in theory how to carry it out.

Let us look carefully at the drawings and the technique outlined in them, and, as usual, move on to their formal training.

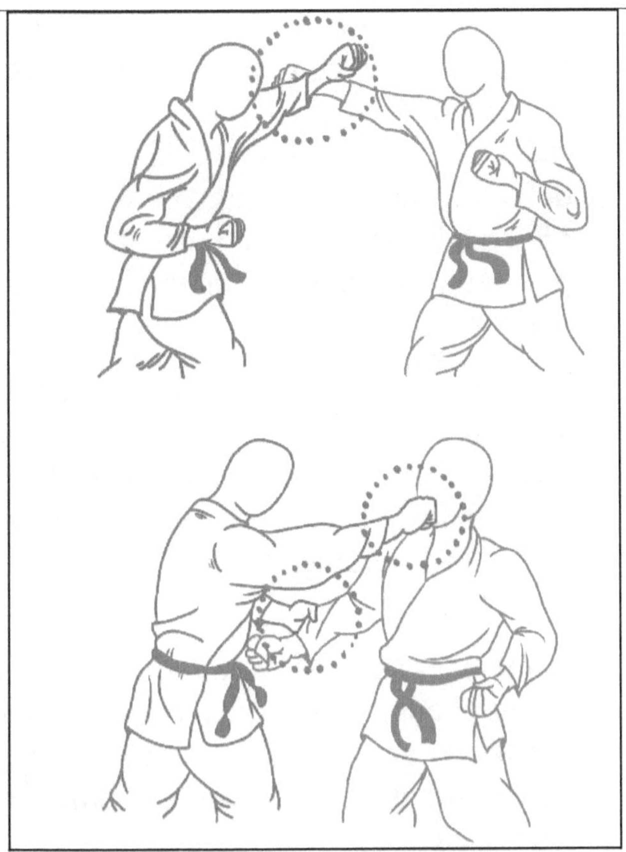

For this, as in all cases, we will try to alternate the practice with companions of all sizes, of different reflections, and if possible, on all kinds of terrain: passengers, rough, wet, etc., in order to thus become a true expert.

My indications are the same as the previous chapter regarding the block of the jab or long left hook. As for our strike with the right arm, I consider that by now the reader will have it well done enough, thoroughly trained, with his hardened fist, accurate aim and a devastating punch.

Well, when blocking the blow, seek to take off balance, on the contrary, take advantage of that fraction of seconds to throw a blow with all the rudeness possible, this if it is a true personal defense, since in training you will have to mark only the blow , without hurting, because what is pursued is a healthy training without injuring the partner.

It is very convenient to practice these casts in the shade to gain speed; Also, use the mirror so that your self-criticism helps you correct any positional vices that you may have acquired in these never-ending trainings if you want to become a virtuoso.

Remember also that with a true enemy in front, things change and you have to be well prepared physically and mentally, in order to be successful at all times, this can only be achieved with tireless practice.

Defensive blocking and lightning offense

Now we will go on to study the new graph, in which a series of three pairs of figures appears that illustrates a lightning attack using four classic karate blows.

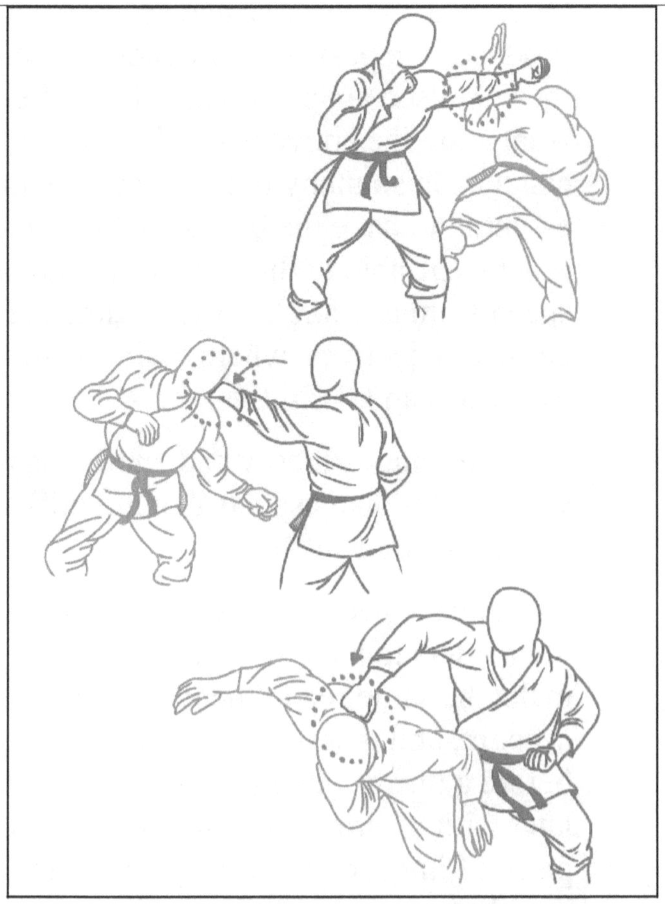

In the first one, that is, the top one, the figure is drawn blocking a jab with a cut, roughly hitting the opponent's knee with a kick. In the second group, a slash blow is illustrated against the opponent's ear, applying said blow diagonally; Finally, in the third illustration, which is the bottom one, a blow with a closed fist against the base of the skull can be seen, thus ending a lightning offensive of four karate blows.

Of course, the surprise and speed aspect is what produces the positive dividends, especially when they are used against laymen in the field. Analyzing the above, we will come to the conclusion so many times discussed, that it is essential to have the blows well executed, in order to be able to throw them with maximum speed from any angle, always aimed at perfectly defined objectives, where their ravages are disastrous and definitive.

But one thing is theory and another is practice, where emotional aspects that are difficult to overcome are shuffled.

Therefore, to achieve the success that I want all my readers to have within this activity, I will make the same recommendation for a new account, and that is to practice tirelessly, first before a mirror, then with shadow exercises and later with a partner, seeking to point out only the place of impact, but already before the natural mobility that a real opponent gives; finally against the sack, where we will unload all the fiber of our blows seeking to achieve effective impacts that indicate the strength that is being capitalized day by day training after training.

At this point the reader will notice that his repertoire has become more formal, that his knowledge is more digested and his ability as a virile Karate performer is becoming more and more noticeable; it is then and not before, when you can start talking about knowing something about this sport.

Defense against a throat attack

In the drawings of the graph, an attack on our throat and the way to get rid of it is illustrated, automatically turning us from attacked into attackers.

For practice, let us study carefully the upper figures, in which the direct attack on our neck appears.

Well, let us, on the contrary, which in this case is our training partner, make contact with our throat, marking the touch so that we can immediately apply the counter, which is the one that appears drawn in the figures below.

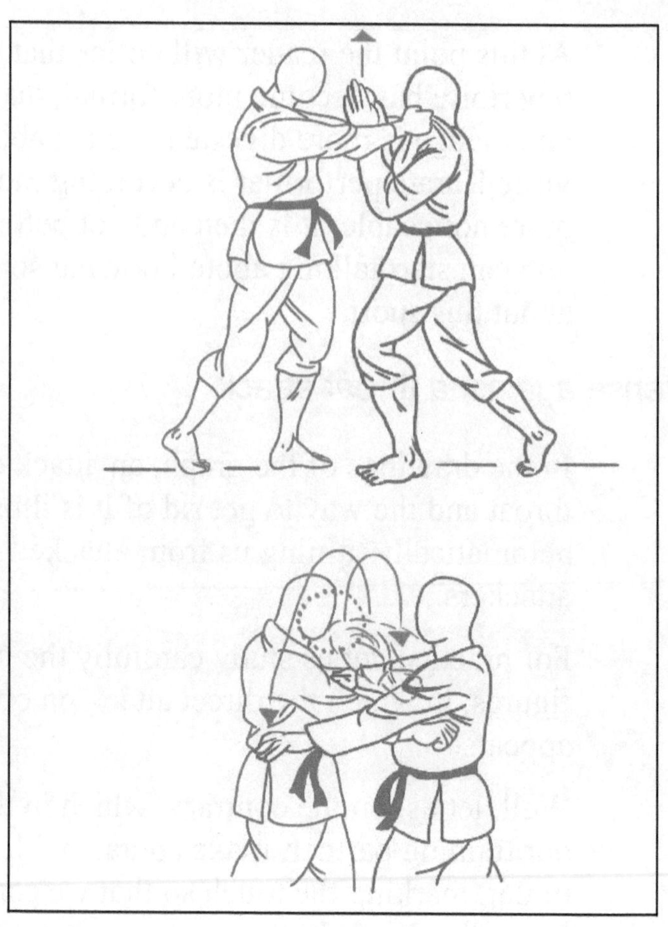

The rule to follow is the following: Bring your palms together at the height of your chest, the tips of your fingers should point up; From this starting position, give a sharp push with your arms, with all your strength, following the direction of the tips of your fingers, that is, upwards; raise your hands to the height of the maximum extension of your arms, when you reach the top open your arms and let your forearms fall roughly on those of your opponent; With the above, the defense is completely finished, the attack was neutralized and we are in a position to immediately attack with karate blows to the head of our opponent.

This blow can be applied with the hand, or with the elbow or both.

We must continue our attack at that moment so that the opponent's moment of weakness is more intelligently used; remember the reader to synchronize the cry of karate that we have talked about earlier at all times, since the confusion brought about by the loud scream is joined by the sequence of strong movements and heavy blows, with which any possible reaction from our opponent will be thwarted .

For the training of this cast, I recommend
alternating with the practice partner, from
attacker to attacked and vice versa, of course
changing as much as possible, the angles of
attack and the places of the attack, so that we can
give the exact counter. anywhere, from the angle
or position in which we find ourselves, however
illogical it may be; for example, hitting with
your back to the wall, knocked down on the
ground, etc.

So, let's train this set conscientiously and go
through the chapter, having it perfectly well
assimilated.

Defense against a blow aimed at the head

In this chapter we will study the way to defend
ourselves from an attack directed against our
head with some blunt object; This type of attack
is very common, hence it is worth doing it
extensively, in order to be prepared to
successfully counter it, as in all the actions that
appear in this treaty, to emerge gracefully
converted from attacked into attackers.

Let's get into the matter by carefully observing the graph, in which an attack is drawn, which we will stop by following the following movements to the letter: Apply slash against the opponent's wrist, as indicated in the corresponding drawing, turn your head as more possible towards the opposite side, to protect it from the possible impact; with the cut the blow stops abruptly, at the same time that we hurt the attacker's hand; Immediately afterwards, we will advance the right foot, as shown in the lower graph, so that it is on the back of the opponent's right leg; in that position apply the karate blow with your heel, so as to hurt his leg and make him lose his balance at the same time; synchronize the previous movements with that of firmly grasping the opponent's wrist and hand,

Look carefully at the way this is done, as with that motif it is shown in the drawing; finish knocking down, on the contrary, making a semicircle movement, which will be described from right to left, thanks to an oscillatory movement of the waist, with which we will help to throw off balance the opponent, who will fall with great ease, without us having to make greater force.

The success of the above lies in the exact positioning of your body, in a sharp and strong blow with your right heel, followed by a push and in the movement of the waist of half circle that is described, all this done at the same time of the grip and twist of the attacking hand.

I repeat this last part.

First is the slash blow, followed by a grip with the same hand to the wrist finished off with a twisting pull that we will do with our right hand, precisely behind the opponent's arm, with which it is solidly secured to our direction; It is necessary to practice the detailed movements in the shadow, doing them in slow motion to accurately locate the places where they are applied, as well as the objective with which the drill is made.

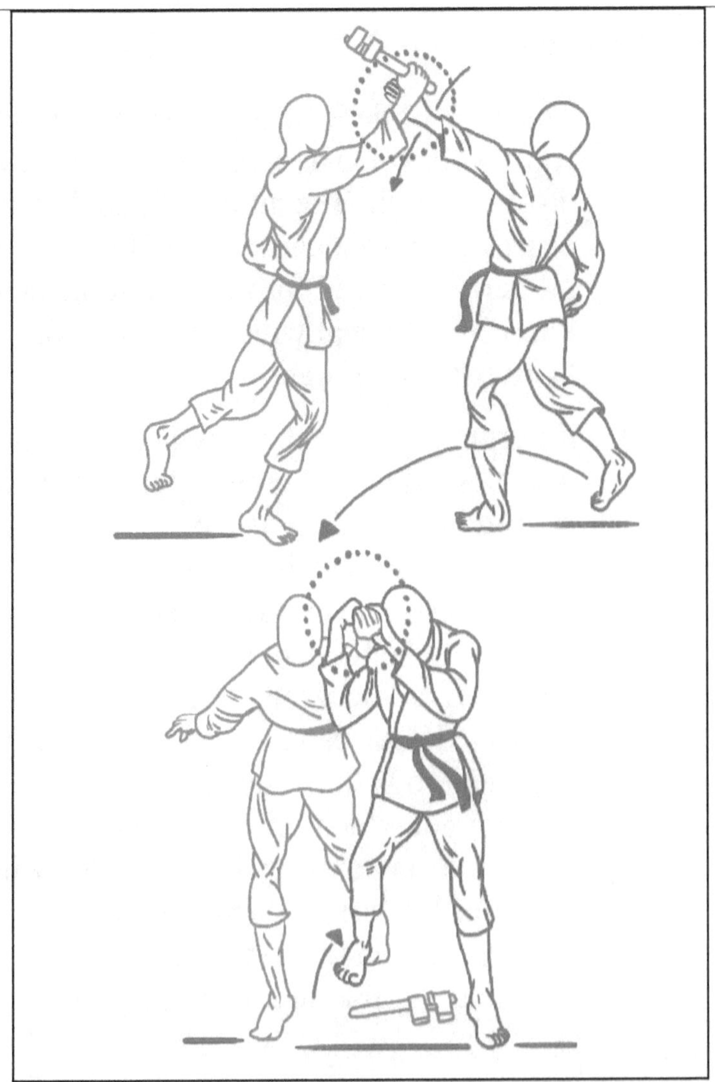

In the first days they will use a soft material, rubber or something similar; When the practice has been understood, it will be carried out with a real object, to learn about reality how to neutralize this attack.

Defense against a boxer

This type of defense is the most necessary to learn well, since in practice this attack is the most common. The attack of people with more or less extensive knowledge of the technique are properly prepared for these contingencies and know how to deal with them using our knowledge of Karate.

Entering the subject, we will go on to study the graph, in which a figure appears throwing the boxing blow known as jab, which is blocked with a strong slash blow to his wrist, which is more effective because at his own strength , the one that the opponent prints with his arm; the block, when blocking, deflects the impact of the jab outside our danger area and forces the opponent to solidly support his left foot against the ground, which gives us the opportunity to apply a strong and dry kick, precisely in the center of his knee; When this blow is given in that place, with the necessary force and aim, it produces the fracture of the patella.

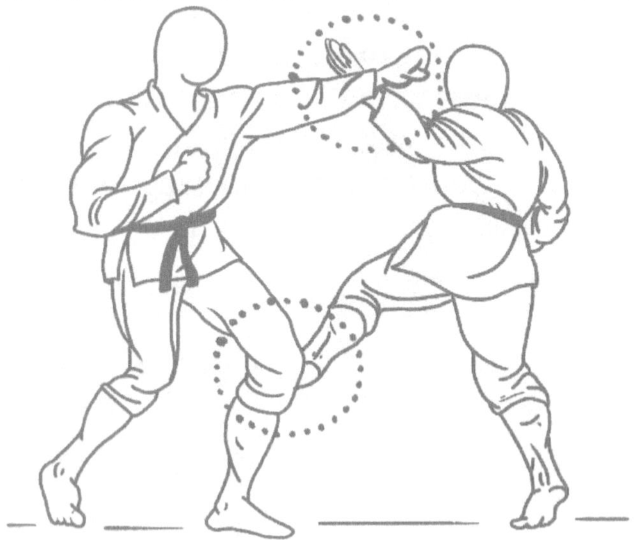

As the reader will be able to appreciate, our knowledge is intensely rude, superior and effective to that of any layman, but in order to render the desired dividend, it must be perfectly executed, that is, it must be carried out strongly, rudely, with our aim and toughness, amen. not to lose balance, which would be counterproductive in their interests.

A fundamental aspect of this set is not to telegraph the intentions with our eyes; because our objective should not be seen directly.

As I have said before, you just have to sidestep and strike unexpectedly.

With the foregoing indications, we will move to the training mat and begin the practice of this cast as many times as necessary until we get it into our blood and we can do it as a reflex, with safety, accuracy and decision.

To fix the exact position, we will start with training exercises in front of the mirror; From there we will go on to shadow exercises, with increasing accuracy; Finally, the practice will be against a partner, looking for precision, but taking care not to hurt.

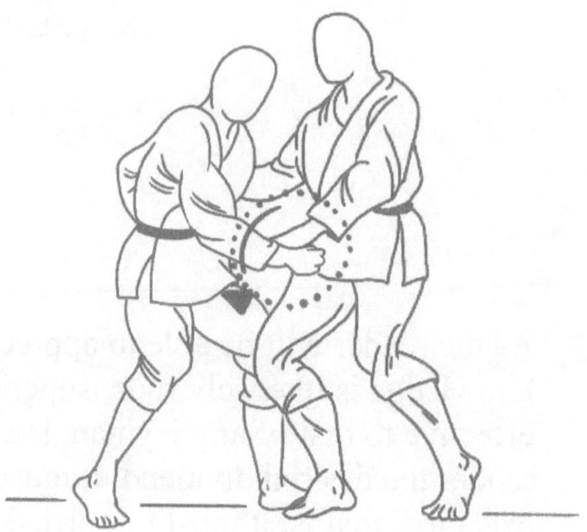

The training bag and constant practice will give us the necessary aim and toughness over time.

Now we will go on to know how to neutralize a boxing blow known as a hook, studying the graph, in which the impact that the cut produces when it hits the opponent's forearm at the moment it is supposed to attack us with a hook is illustrated right.

From our guard position, it comes out with sharp speed and forces the cut that blocks said blow, diverting it out of our body; the slash gains strength when making contact, because at one to our movement the strength of the opponent, turning it into a blow receiving very forceful.

In this case, the gap that the cut creates momentarily must be used to attack with one or more karate blows against the opponent's face.

It is necessary to mention the rudeness that cutting blows can acquire when the hand is strong enough; Between nothing and with adequate malice, any forearm can be fractured with relative ease, but of course, a layman would not achieve that, since, to obtain such results, constant practice of many years is necessary in order to harden the hand in such a way that his slash strokes invariably fracture when counting.

So, let's practice first in front of the necessary mirror, then with shadow exercises, and finally, against our partner, at the same time that we continue to harden our hands with the daily practice of cutting, hitting a board, as indicated in the corresponding chapter.

Defense against a slap

In the graph, the way to counteract a slap is drawn, which is blocked before reaching its destination, using his arm to punish his daring.

Let's first study the theory of drawing before moving on to its formal training.

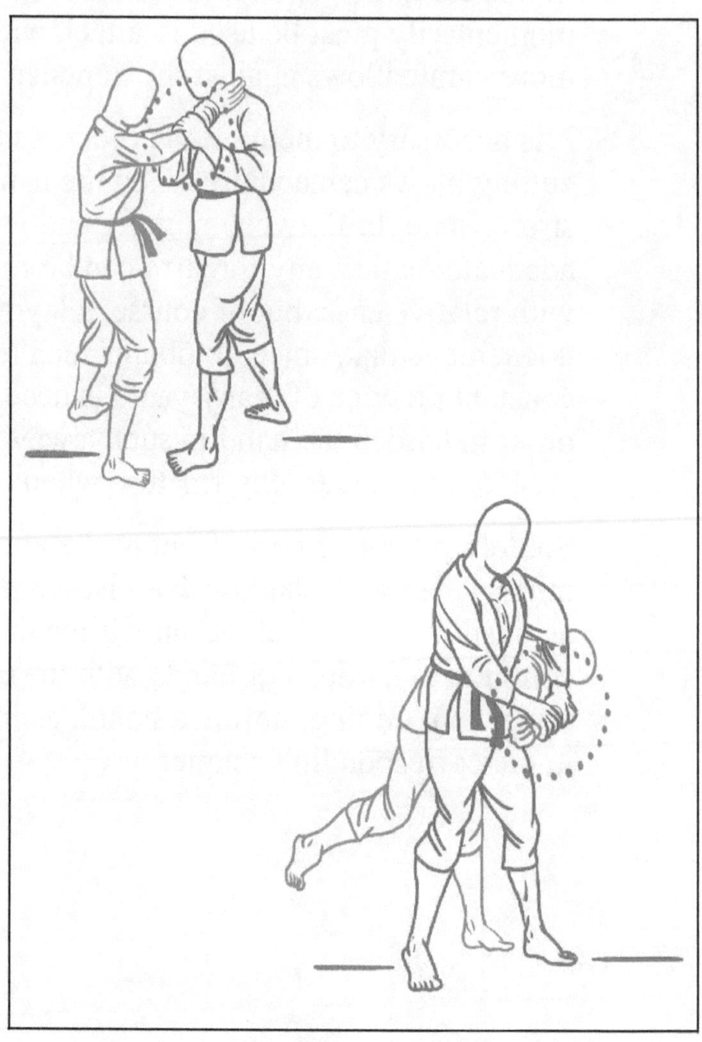

Note that the blocking of the opponent's right hand is done by catching his wrist with our right hand, grasping it completely with the left; to prevent it from coming loose when it is properly secured, proceed to make a half turn on your left leg, so as to stay in the position indicated in the drawings in the lower illustration; Keep the opponent's wrist strongly secured, so that when reaching the indicated position, it is said movement that strongly harasses the opponent's elbow, which will be at our mercy, pointing the movement upwards, so that any pressure from us towards down, may cause the immediate fracture of it.

Use your left elbow to hit the opponent's temple, preventing it from slipping away; when the reader is the one who has fallen in this set, use the counter that consists of arching the elbow to avoid being pried against it, seek to crouch as much as possible and with the left hand, imprison the ankle of the opposite of the same side; Push your shoulder forward, jerk your pinched ankle down.

This blockade is extremely simple, it actually leaves our sport to invade a bit of wrestling, but it is advisable for my readers to know all the resources.

That is precisely why I have not hesitated one iota to include it in their repertoire. Well, we have already analyzed this set in its theoretical aspect, so that it is time to transfer its knowledge and functions to the practical aspect of its formal training, that is, against an opponent.

Look for the first few occasions to do it in slow motion, in order to find the exact touch that leads to the place where the punishment occurs and the way to counter; When the above has been achieved well, we will move on to the speed in execution aspect, alternating with the training partner, sometimes as an attacker, sometimes as an attacked, in order to familiarize ourselves as necessary with this set.

My recommendation is that the reader for no reason goes to another chapter without first having this perfectly mastered.

Defense against a head attack

In the graph, a fairly common attack is illustrated; It is an attack against the head with any object that has more or less the drawn shape.

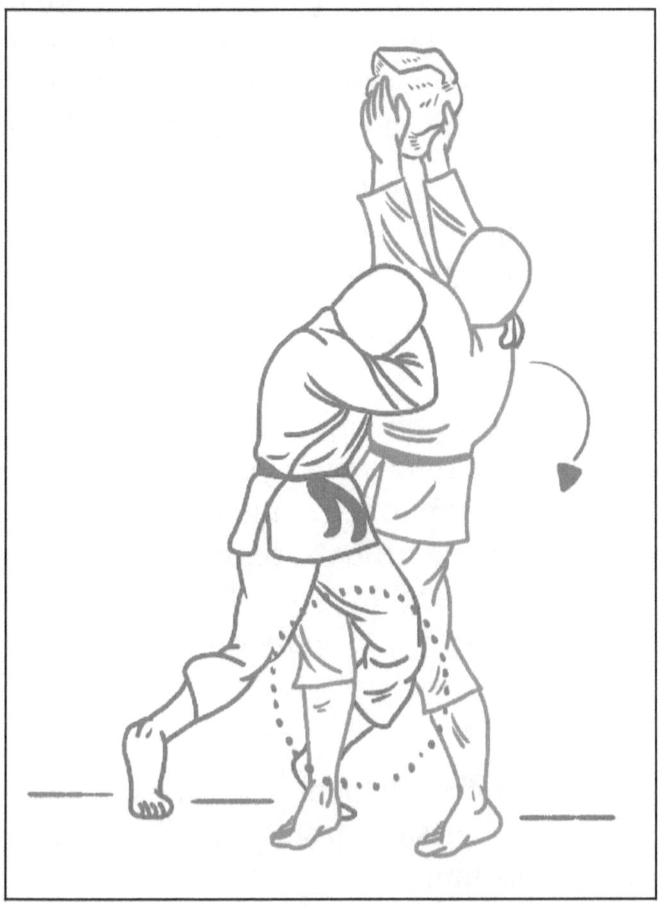

In this chapter we will study how to defend ourselves wisely by using our knowledge of karate to counterattack. To do this, the reader must carefully observe the drawing where the way to neutralize the attack can be seen, which consists of getting ahead of the opponent and, before it can make an impact, control it at the moment in which he telegraphed his intention by raising his threatening arms with the stone.

Then we will launch ourselves with the greatest possible speed to embrace his arms, advancing our head next to his, in order to remove it from the focus of aggression, thereby avoiding danger.

Squeeze your arms, stick your head to your body, strongly push your attacker to the front, tilting him to the left in a semicircle movement, to get him off balance, making him lose his balance slightly, an instant that we will take advantage of to apply a strong trip against his left leg, using our leg on the same side, which will make the attacker fall easily.

When this happens, use karate blows with your feet, knees and hands, in order to definitively break him.

Let the reader practice this way of succeeding in this dangerous set, training with his companions, using a soft object the first few times, which can be a pillow, in order to avoid unnecessary injuries in the learning process.

As we progress in the control and clean execution of the cast, we will change the cushion for a sturdier object, doing the training more thoroughly. Finally, the training will be done with a heavy object, of course being careful not to hurt yourself.

The idea is to accustom the reader to effectively control his nerves in the face of real danger, focusing on a ground of absolute truthfulness so as not to be intimidated when it is necessary to face a risk of this nature in everyday life.

The training should be done alternating with the partner (s), sometimes as an attacker, other times as an attacked, until this throw is controlled.

Lastly, I recommend getting ahead of the attacker with speed and malice.

Defense against an attack a dagger

In the following graphic, they are presented with three figures, a dagger attack. It presents the way to counterattack using karate blows coupled with knowledge of personal defense.

So, let's take a closer look at the figures and for your practical learning, let's move on to the training mat.

I suggest that, to avoid unnecessary injuries, a rubber or plastic dagger is used during training. The way to control this attack is as follows: He appears placed in a guard position, with his hands ready to strike with Tagus; When the attack occurs, hit the opponent's forearm hard with said blow, closest to his hand, so the cut will stop the possible stab; In that very small interval, we will make the following movements, also in a fraction of a second: First, we will apply a poke blow against his eyes with the fingers of our hand in a V shape, we will advance our right leg and with our right arm we will hold the opposite one to the height of about three centimeters above your elbow, with our left hand, that after the blow, the armed arm will have been detaining outwards; we will make an outward folding movement, so that the opposite is placed in the position illustrated in the central drawings; already placed in this situation, we are the ones who have the advantage, because with a strong blow with the arch of our right foot on his calf on the same side, we will make him fall; When we fall to our knees, we will raise our armed arm, with which the shoulder can be dislocated, causing enough pain, so that we immediately drop the weapon, thus remaining at our entire disposal. we are the ones who have the advantage, because with a strong blow with the arch of our right foot on his calf on the same side, we will make him fall; When we fall to our knees, we will raise our armed arm, with which the shoulder can be dislocated, causing enough pain, so that we immediately drop the weapon, thus remaining at our entire disposal. we are the ones who have the advantage, because with a strong blow with the arch of our right foot on his calf on the same side, we will make him fall; When we fall to our knees, we will raise our armed arm, with which the shoulder can be dislocated, causing enough pain, so that we immediately drop the weapon, thus remaining at our entire disposal.

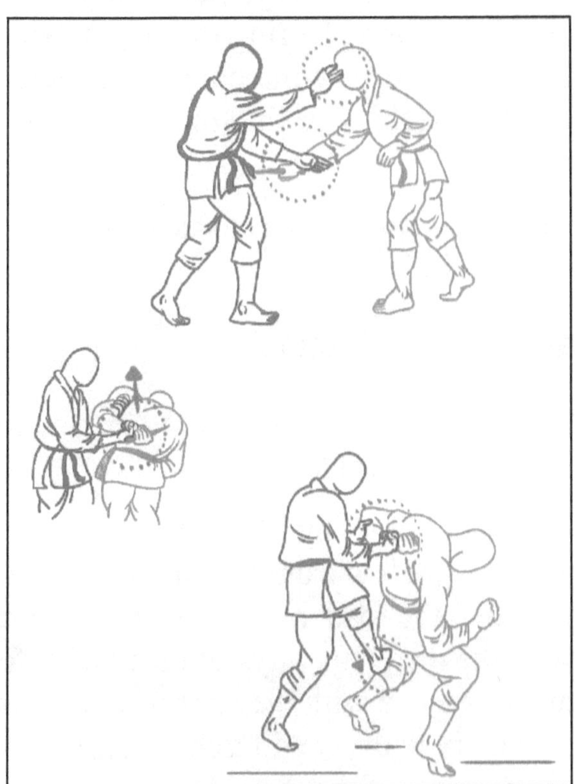

In order to capture the above, it is necessary to read it thoroughly and practice it exhaustively on the training mat, with the partner in front, in slow motion, both in common agreement, go step by step learning the development of the present cast, otherwise their learning will not be possible.

The success of this cast lies in two aspects: in the speed with which the cut to the armed forearm and the stab to the eyes were applied simultaneously; During training sessions, the sting in the eyes will be marked, decisively and quickly, seeking to find the exact touch of this throw.

Train it as many times as necessary, until it is fully assimilated.

Defense against a stab attack

In the graph, we present another way to counter a stabbing attack.

The upper drawing illustrates the shape of the attack, which is from bottom to top and in front; By now, the reader will have become familiar with the different ways of using a knife to attack, and of course with the appropriate cons for each special type of wielding the weapon; Well, this is apparently the most dangerous, so it will be the one that we will study more carefully.

In theory, the ideal way to counter is by standing in our guard position, with your hands ready for the chop.

Wait quietly for the onslaught; when this happens, arch your body so as to remove the bundle and with a strong blow, grasp the armed hand firmly; of a quick turn of half a turn, keeping the opponent's hand secured, directing the danger out of her body, turning the back of the opponent; Raise the arm of your enemy, apply the key known in wrestling as Marcus's lever, which consists of placing the opponent's elbow on our right shoulder and making a strong lever movement with the shoulder up, with our hands to the opposite side, that is, downwards, rudely punishing the opponent's elbow, so that he lets go of the weapon before the alternative that with the aforementioned Marcus lever we break his arm, disarticulating it at the elbow.

The pain is so strong when the key is properly applied that it will immediately make you drop the gun and give up.

Now we will go from theory to practice on the mattress and with the indispensable training partner. The first shots will be taken in slow motion, looking for the exact place to punish without being hurt; When you find the ideal touch, as we sportly call the place of punishment, we will have taken the first step and we will only lack speed, which is obtained by practicing tirelessly, changing partners so as not to get used to a single individual, since this is harmful; try to alternate your practice with partners of different reflexes, sizes, etc., seeking to execute this cast as cleanly as possible.

I recommend using a soft rubber plastic knife for practice; When you are an expert, use a real dagger, but this, as I indicated before, will be when you are already an expert, before your results can be counterproductive.

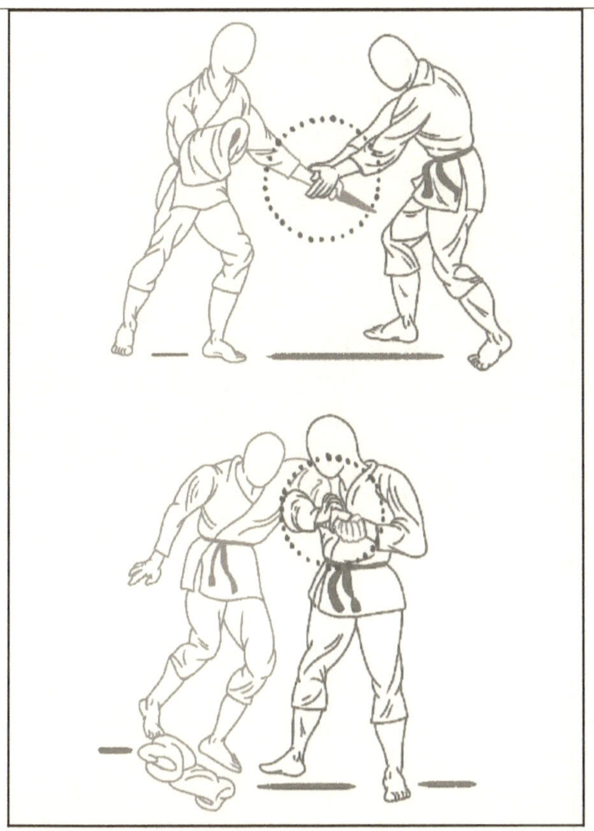

Defense against a blow to the head

In this chapter we will learn to stop a blow against our head using our arms in the shape of a cross, as indicated in the graph, in which an attack with the handle of a pistol appears.

The ideal way to stop this blow by forming a cross with your arms over your head, holding your fists closed.

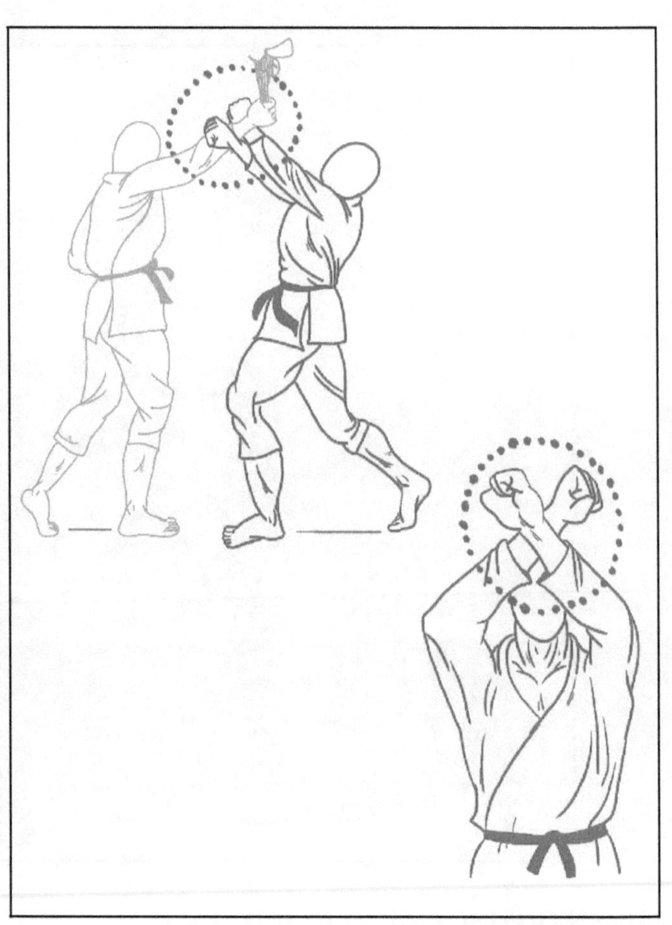

When stopping the blow, the opponent's forearm is imprisoned in the cross that ours will form. This movement is apparently easy to achieve, but it is not in reality since it requires exact muscular coordination and vision of the place to exactly catch the blow before it reaches its destination; When stopping said blow, immediately open your hands firmly grasping the armed arm, seeking to quickly apply the counter based on karate blows, either an elbow, or a blow with the knee in the place where the sex is located, to punish the attacker harshly forcing him to let go of the arm by giving up his offense, or by making a full half turn with his right leg, so as to turn his back on him, but keeping the armed arm firmly imprisoned.

At the end of this turn, the simple movement will cause him to fall into a punishment grip, which will increase if we increase our pressure against his arm, turning him so that his elbow is pointing up and we punishing down, to cause the pain on the contrary. necessary in order for him to drop his weapon and surrender.

In theory, the above seems straightforward. To make it effective, we need to train it many times, suggesting that a toy gun made of plastic or rubber material be used for its training; when their learning has been achieved, we can use a more forceful object; If a real pistol is used, we must be careful to examine well that it is unloaded.

In training I always demand a lot of caution to avoid unnecessary injuries, since what is sought is a white, sporty and healthy training, tending to make the reader an expert in self-defense.

Therefore, once again I recommend that the practices be carried out intelligently, with due prudence.

Defense against a feint head on, with a pistol

Now we will study how to get out of a gun threat, which is illustrated in the graph, as well as how to get out of it. Well, supposing that we are threatened, as is classic with our hands up, the basic thing is to keep cool blood, calm, controlled nerves, our attentive eyes, watching those of the opposite, trying to guess their possible mistakes.

The counter consists of lowering the arms like lightning, grasping the armed hand with our left hand, deflecting the barrel of the pistol away from the target that our body presents; With the right hand we will give a strong slap on the barrel of the same, securing it firmly, attacking against the weak part of the hand that in this case is represented by its thumb; The movement will be taking the barrel of the gun secured, first towards the right side, attacking the thumb, then with force, downwards, taking into account that with the right hand we will have firmly secured its wrist and we will lift it upwards, so that apply force to the opposite side of the right hand, with this we will be able to disarm it easily.

He then counterattacks with an elbow, if he is close to us, if he is not, we will hit him on the head with the handle of his pistol; This cast seems simple, its nerve is in the speed with which we grasp his right hand with our left, diverting the aim and the skill and force with which we attack the cannon with the right hand, which is the most skilled.

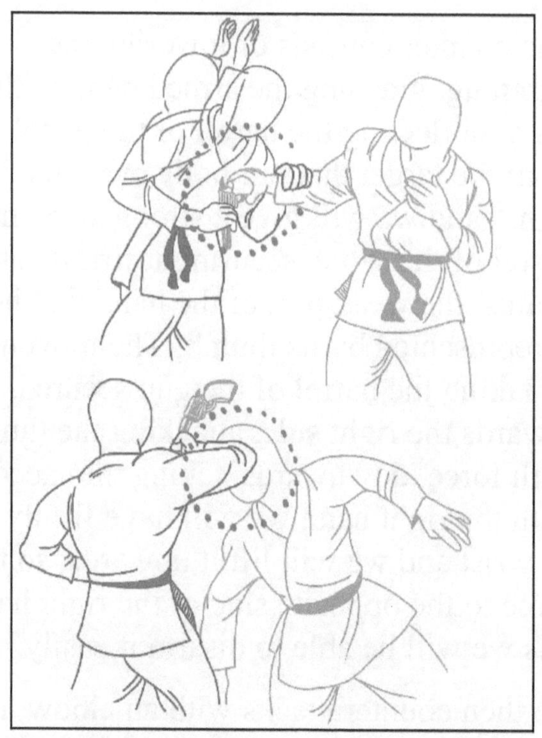

Now, after the previous theory, let's move on to practice, which should be done with a toy gun that will be triggered so that the student can confront whether his movements were fast enough to avoid an outcome against him.

Switch with your partner from attacker to attacker, in order to liven up the training somewhat, and do not change chapters until you have fully learned this interesting means of personal defense.

If you use a real pistol in your practice, I suggest checking carefully before it is unloaded.

Defense against a feint from behind, with a pistol

Continuing on in our self-defense learning, we will go on to study the graph, in which a pistol attack is illustrated in which we are with our hands up, as is classic, pointed at the back.

The way to get out of this quagmire is as follows: Locate by touch the height where the gun that threatens you is, that is, feel where it is, in what part of your body.

As in all cases, I recommend control of your nerves, speed, decision and agility.

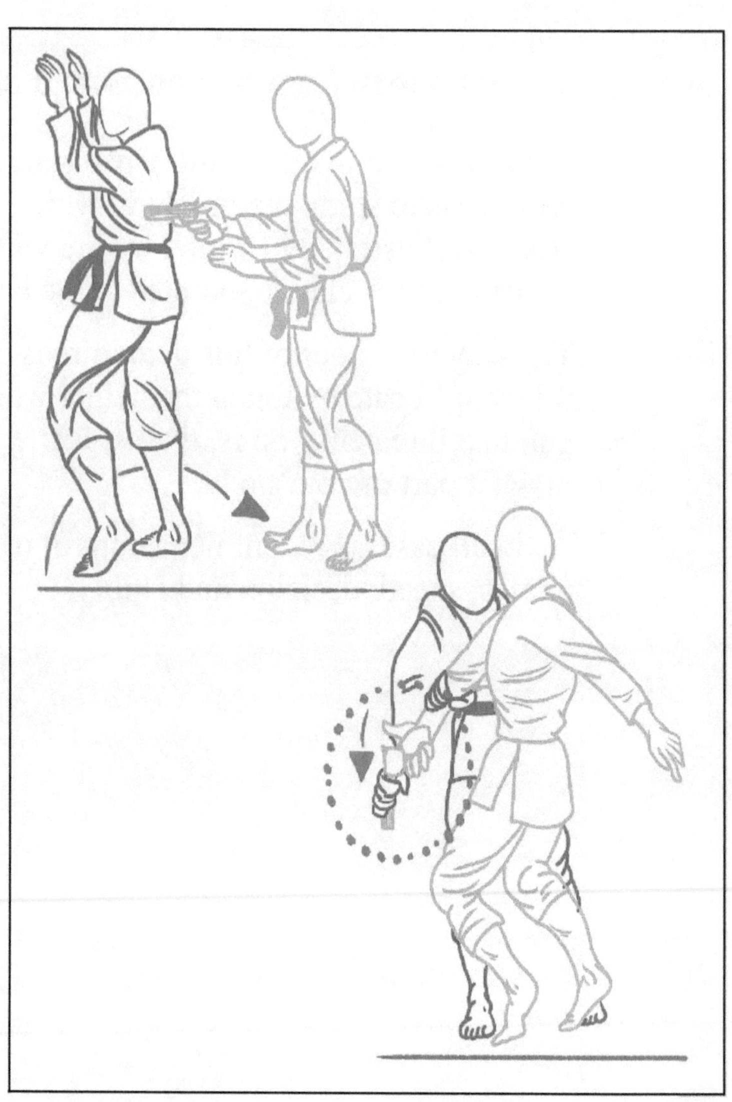

Make a very rapid turn as indicated in the graph, turn around so that with that turn you remove your body from the target it presented; immediately attack the armed arm, imprisoning it with the left hand at the wrist; in one position it will direct the danger of the weapon to the other side; With your right hand, cache the barrel of the pistol and with the firmly secured, make two strong and definitive movements, one towards the thumb, attacking it, since this part represents the weak part of the hand; subsequently with a strong downward pull, thereby disarming the attacker; immediately the situation is in their hands.

Proceed to punish harshly with karate blows with your elbows or with the handle of the pistol that will now be in your right hand.

The development of the previous cast is necessary to put it into practice on the training mat, in order to assimilate it, understand it and find where its exact touch is.

For your training I recommend using a toy gun, loaded with caps, which the partner will trigger so that the reader knows if he was able to get out of the attack in a timely manner, or if the result was negative.

Similarly, a water gun is used to visualize a path.

As training allows everything, we can gradually see if we progress or not in our knowledge; The first few times the practice will be in slow motion, carefully marking the movements, seeking more than the sporty aspect, to perfectly coordinate the ideal counter.

In later practices, having well learned the turns and grip locations, we will seek to obtain speed and effectiveness.

Before going on to another chapter, convince yourself if you have mastered this set perfectly; if so, we can move on; if not, we will practice exhaustively as many times as necessary, until we reach perfection. Take into account that your life will be involved if you ever find yourself in this situation, without having control of the counter that we deal with in this chapter.

Defense against kicks using the slash

Now we will study how to use the slash to neutralize a kick. To do this, we will observe the graph, in which the way to attack by defending is illustrated.

Observe the reader the place where a forceful cut is applied, which at the same time as for the impact of the kick, hurts strongly, since our target is the opponent's shin, an extremely vulnerable and painful place.

In the chapter referring to the study of the cut, I present in detail how to harden the hands, preparing them to strike with the edge of the same heavy blows. On this occasion we have the opportunity to practice the knowledge learned from a completely different angle to the known ones, but no less interesting to master, hence we practice as many times as necessary to achieve a strong and devastating cut, which when applied pays two dividends simultaneously, defend ourselves and hurt.

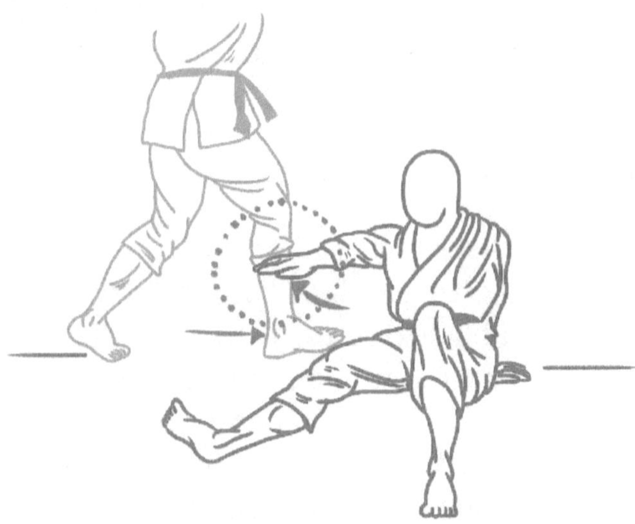

My recommendation, as in all cases, is to practice as much as necessary until its complete assimilation, taking care to execute your slash stroke well, hitting exactly with the hand, not with the fingers, as it would run the risk of hurting them, since These are weak compared to the shin on the attacker's leg, but if his hand is well hardened and his cut perfectly learned, the risk I am referring to will be negligible.

Let's take advantage of this chapter to insist once again on the conscientious training of the pit, which by now should have the reader perfectly executed; If not, go back and train as necessary to fully master the resource in question.

Defense against an attack by two individuals

Attacks by criminals who use the wrestling key known as "China" for their misdeeds have been published so many times in the newspapers that I have not resisted the temptation to present to the readers of this modest treatise, the form of defense to This type of immoral assault, in which one of the criminals entertains the future victim from the front, while the other ruffian quietly stands behind behind him and attacks with the aforementioned key to the throat, a key that in most cases leads to death.

Well, the way to get out of a situation like the one mentioned more or less well is by using your karate knowledge intelligently, in the following way (see next graphic): First, you ruthlessly hit the testicles of the ruffian in front of you with your leg. preferably using the heel of the foot; if the blow is delivered with the accurate aim that my readers will have or should have by now, the result will be that the first will immediately abandon the fight.

Then proceed to give the counter key, putting your hands inside the knot that forms the attacker's arm, pushing with their palms to the front and to the sides, with all the force that is possible, to loosen the dangerous tie It attacks your apple or Adam's apple.

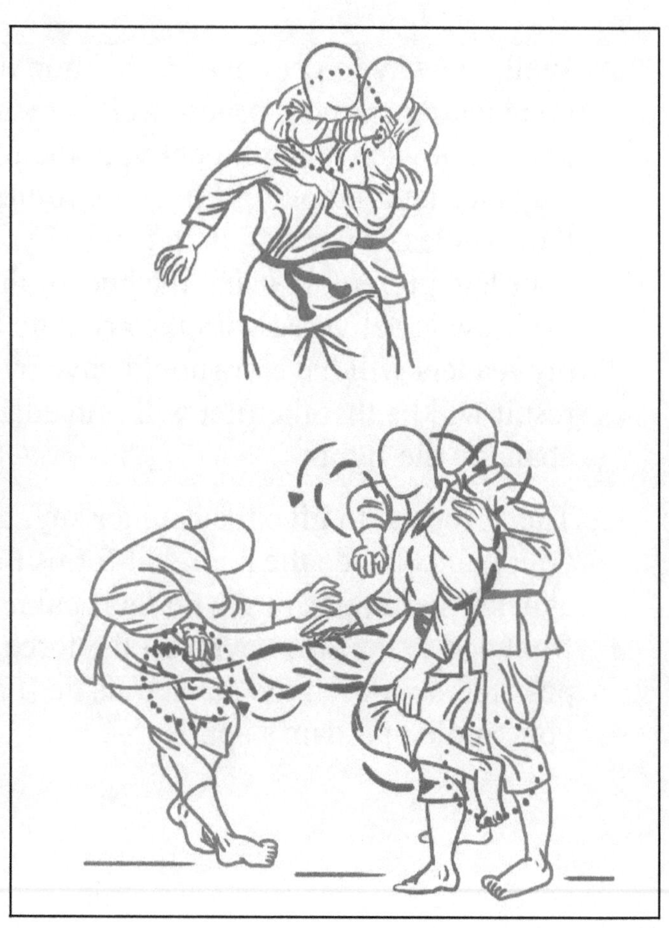

In order to protect it, turn your neck sharply to the left, in order to get it out of danger, hit the attacker's face with your skull and always move forward to throw the opponent off balance; When you manage to loosen the knot that closes against your throat, use another karate device that is to hit the opponent's shin or knee with the heel, punishing him with force; This blow must be strong, surprising, to take the enemy off balance, using as usual in a katarista, the fractions of seconds that the surprise of unforeseen, unknown blows gives us, to finish freeing ourselves from the threat to our throat and apply a ruthless elbow against the face of the former attacker, who from that second will be at our mercy and at our entire disposal.

I recommend practicing this cast to a superlative degree, which can be very useful in everyday life, as long as it is well mastered; For this, exhaustive practice on the mattress will be the guideline to follow. Train with your training partner, first in slow motion, then only by dialing and finally do your roughest workouts with the idea of obtaining the necessary blank, but always without failing to observe due caution.

First aid

In all sports some mishaps tend to happen from time to time, ours could by no means be the exception, since in it certain rough hauls are executed, emanating from its own rudeness, however, the cautious prudence with which I demand be carried to effect their practices; but these accidents do not involve serious danger in strong individuals, with good physical preparation.

Therefore, in this chapter we will study what these contingencies may be and how to administer first aid while the doctor arrives.

Even so, it is equally advisable to have the treatise "The Dragon's Health Philosophy".

The most common accidents are:

Nosebleeds. This problem is very common among aspirants, being it advisable in such cases to apply cold compresses to the base of the nose, forehead and neck, in addition to tapping with a cotton pad soaked with adrenaline (anesthetic) on the affected part.

KO for hit to the head. When this happens, give the casualty artificial respiration, inhale aromatic salts or ammonia; shelter it as well as possible and put it to rest. When the applicant is in good physical condition, the above has no consequences; But, anyway, you should rest for a week, abstaining from hard training, and it is advisable to have it checked by a doctor.

Bone fracture. The appropriate thing in these cases is the absolute immobility of the affected part, putting the injured person comfortable, warm in perfect rest, if it is possible to apply mud, mud, sand or thermal clay in the affected area and immediately call a doctor, or the relatives for their safe transfer.

Cut in the face. These annoying accidents tend to happen very often when one head is hit against another, producing annoying and bulky cuts; in this case it is advisable to rub the wounds with a cotton pad soaked in adrenaline, and apply a thick layer of thermal mud, or pure solid petroleum jelly, mixed with surgical sulfathiazole powder, or elastic collodion; if the case warrants it, go to the doctor to put the necessary stitches.

Purple eyes. This accident is the most common and simple; It is recommended to apply compresses of cold water and thermal mud in order to make the bruise disappear.

Dislocations. This problem is extremely annoying, especially when there are muscle or tendon tears; of course it is rare in athletes with good preparation, but in the end an accident, which gets out of control and usually happens; When this happens, put the injured person at rest, gently sell the affected part with an elastic bandage and see that an expert in these tasks intervenes; don't try to massage if you don't know exactly what to do. The injured person must rest long enough before a new training session.

KO for hit to the bass. This happens with some frequency, but it is not dangerous later; It is recommended to give artificial respiration to the injured person, apply oxygen if you have it on hand, wrap him well and let him rest, nature takes care of the rest.

My recommendation is not to underestimate any of these problems, nor to give it more emphasis than necessary.

The listed contingencies can be avoided with good prudence. The strong physical condition that is obtained by carrying out more recommendations, of training and preparing first with the exercises presented in the relative chapters, avoid annoying accidents in a high percentage of the time, since your body will be strong and resistant. But of course, we must not confuse machismo with what caution advises.

This work was finished on September 2, 2020 in Mexico City, being published by the same author under his own publishing brand "Zone Black".

More from the author:

1. The Dragon's health philosophy
2. Lifestyles (drawing manual)
3. Leonardo Gudiño's combat method
4. The tao of drawing
5. The great newfoundland
6. The Art of War Unveiled
7. Dynamic line (drawing manual)
8. Multiverses other realities
9. Area 51
10. Attitude in drawings

www.ingramcontent.com/pod-product-compliance
Lightning Source LLC
Chambersburg PA
CBHW051452250726
48655CB00001B/366